Springer Series on Social Work
Albert R. Roberts, D.S.W., Series Editor
Graduate School of Social Work, Rutgers, The State University of New Jersey

Julianne S. Oktay, M.S.W., Ph.D. is an associate professor at the University of Maryland School of Social Work in Baltimore. Dr. Oktay received her undergraduate degree from Antioch College and did her graduate work at the University of Michigan. She has written many books and articles in the field of social work in health care. She is married and has two daughters.

Carolyn Ambler Walter, M.S.S., Ph.D. is a clinical social worker and an assistant professor in the Center for Social Work Education at Widener University in Chester, Pennsylvania. Dr. Walter received her Ph.D, and her M.S.S. at the School of Social Work and Social Research at Bryn Mawr College. Dr. Walter is the author of *The Timing of Motherhood* and other articles pertaining to women's concerns and life-cycle issues. She is married and has two teenaged children.

Breast Cancer in the Life Course
Women's Experiences

Julianne S. Oktay
Carolyn A. Walter

Springer Publishing Company
New York

Springer Publishing Company, Inc.
536 Broadway
New York, NY 10012-3955

91   92   93   94   95 / 5 4 3 2 1

Library of Congress Cataloging-in-Publication Data

Oktay, Julianne S.
    Breast cancer in the life course: women's experiences/Julianne
S. Oktay and Carolyn A. Walter.
      p.   cm.—(Springer series on social work; v. 20)
    Includes bibliographical references and index.
    ISBN 0-8261-7110-9: $28.95 (prepub)
      1. Breast—Cancer—Psychological aspects—Age factors.
I. Walter, Carolyn Ambler. II. Title. III. Series.
RC280,B8037   1990
616.99'449'019—dc20   91-2260
                                                                    CIP

Printed in the United States of America

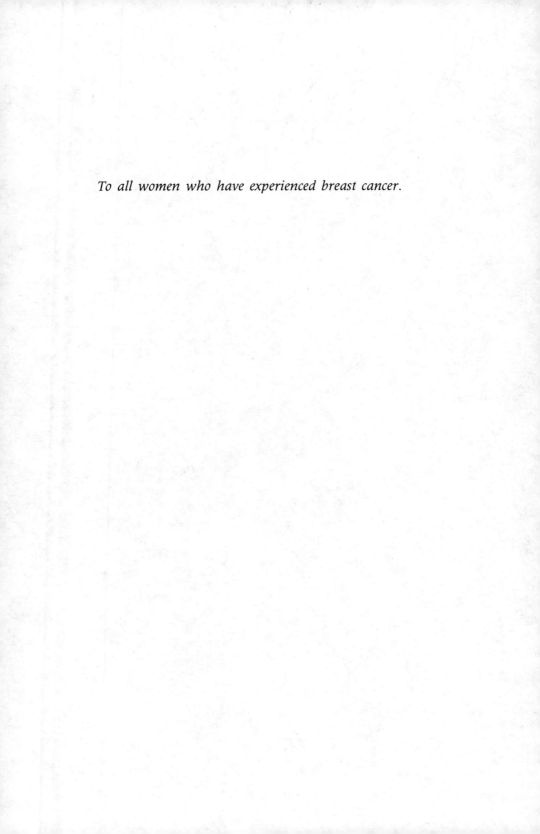

To all women who have experienced breast cancer.

Contents

Acknowledgments

So many people have helped us create this book. First and foremost, the entire project would have been impossible without the forty-two women whose voices make up the heart of this book. Thanks go to them for inspiring us, for so openly sharing with us, and for making us sure of the value of what we were doing. We have tried to preserve the essence of what they wanted to say. We are deeply grateful to them, and apologize for all the wonderful quotes and stories we had to omit, and for whatever we may have been unsuccessful in portraying accurately.

Secondly, we initially decided to work on breast cancer shortly after the death (from breast cancer) of Jane Gibson, a close friend of Carolyn. Jane's experiences got us started on the topic, and throughout the process, her memory and her graceful spirit has powerfully motivated us. In fact, the book was "born" exactly four years after her death. Thanks, Jane!

We thank the chapters of the American Cancer Society that invited us to their meetings and helped us to contact women who had had breast cancer. Thanks too, for referrals, to Sherri Alper, Joan Applegate, Wanda Bair, Paula Dubé, Marcia Martin, Lori Mossberg (Comprehensive Breast Care Center, Cooper Hospital, Camden, NJ), Pam Sorok (William Beaumont Hospital, Royal Oak, MI), and Patti Wilcox (Johns Hopkins Oncology Center, Baltimore, MD).

Both the University of Maryland at Baltimore and Widener University provided funding through faculty research grants.

Marcia Egan and Nadine Shaberman did several excellent interviews, providing us with a broadened perspective on rural and elderly women. Linda Walker and Lori Mossberg edited the manuscript carefully, and also provided both thoughtful criticism and warm encouragement. The book was improved enormously by their input. Thanks, Linda and Lori! Special thanks, too, to Dr. Andrew Dorr, Jr. (National Cancer Institute), Dr. Anne Hahn, and Dr. David Hahn for their valuable comments on earlier versions of chapter 1.

Sarah Fought and Renée Forbes did a wonderful job bringing out the women's voices as they transferred the interviews from the tapes. Gwen Young and Libby Murach put in tireless hours typing the manuscript. Hannah Treitel methodically prepared the references and helped with manuscript preparation.

We are also so appreciative of the support we have received from our families and friends—especially our husbands, who have been continual sources of support, and our parents, who provided us with something so essential to any kind of creativity—a sense of trust and confidence in ourselves.

Introduction

One out of 10 American women is destined to have breast cancer during her lifetime (American Cancer Society, 1990). In 1990, approximately 150,000 American women are estimated to be diagnosed with breast cancer, and about 44,000 will die from the disease. To put these figures in perspective, 57,000 Americans died in the Vietnam war, and, to date, about 60,000 have died from the acquired immunodeficiency disorder (AIDS). This means that almost as many women die from breast cancer *per year* as the total number who have died from AIDS since the epidemic began. About as many women are diagnosed *per year* with breast cancer as have been diagnosed with AIDS in 10 years. Breast cancer is the commonest form of cancer among American women. Despite advances in early detection and treatments, the mortality rate from breast cancer has not changed significantly in the last 50 years. This book is about breast cancer as it is experienced by women of varying ages, from the late 20s to the 70s. Through case studies and short vignettes, women across the life cycle share their experiences with breast cancer.

Although theories of adult development have become popular (Sheehy, 1976) in recent years, these theories have not yet been related systematically to the understanding of adjustment to breast cancer. In an attempt to understand how women of different ages adapt and cope with breast cancer, we have examined how the common tasks necessary for healthy adaptation to breast cancer interact with major life tasks of each phase of adulthood (early adulthood, middle adulthood, and later adulthood). Through women's voices we examine how specific tasks in adjusting to breast cancer are related to life-stage issues faced by the patient and her family.

In this chapter, we point out four traditions that influence our work: adaptation to illness, life-course development, experiencing illness, and women's voices. We then review the methodology of the study including the sample, interviews, analysis, and limitations. Finally, we present an overview of the book.

TRADITIONS

This book builds on several separate "traditions" or areas of thought.

Adaptation to Illness

First is the knowledge of the problems faced by all those going through a serious illness. Psychologists, social workers, and health practitioners have developed conceptualizations of illness experience that involve a common set of "tasks." For example, almost all illness involves some limitation in functioning, and this may necessitate adaptation to shifts in roles. The conceptualizations we have used most heavily in our thinking are those developed by Moos and Tsu (1977) and Mailick (1979). The tasks we have chosen to discuss are those most appropriate to the experience of breast cancer. Those tasks are discussed in detail in chapter 1.

Life-Course Development

Another stream of knowledge that this book uses is life-course development in adulthood. During the last 15 years there has been a heightened interest in adult development theory that makes a valuable contribution because it highlights the "presence and persistence of growth and change" throughout adulthood (Weick, 1983).

There is no single, dominant adult development theory like there is for the childhood and adolescent portions of the life cycle. One reason may be the greater complexity of the adult world "along with a greater variability of individual patterns in dealing with developmental tasks" (Blumberg, Flaherty, & Lewis, 1982, p. 7). Although children encounter similar developmental tasks at about the same chronological age, adults vary in age as to when certain life events occur.

Less is known about women when compared with men regarding early, middle, and later adulthood. Some researchers and writers have agreed that the "lives of women follow different patterns and involve somewhat different themes than do the lives of men" (Reinke, Holmes, & Harris, 1985, p. 1353; Jenks, 1983), yet others see similarities in the adult development of men and women (Levinson, Darrow, Klein, Levinson, &

McKee, 1978; Roberts & Newton, 1987; Stewart, 1977). It has been suggested that women's lives are guided by the development of attachment and care (Chodorow, 1978; Gilligan,1982b; Miller, 1986; Rubin, 1979), whereas men's lives are guided by the development of individuation and autonomy.

Because a comprehensive theory of women's development does not yet exist (Roberts & Newton, 1987), when using life-course theory to understand women's experiences with breast cancer, we have synthesized themes and data from adult development theory and research based on the lives of men (Erikson, 1980; Levinson et al., 1978), the lives of women (Baruch, Barnett, & Rivers, 1983; Gilligan, 1982b; Roberts & Newton, 1987; Rubin, 1979), and the lives of men and women (Gould, 1979; Neugarten, 1968, 1975). Although Erikson's model of adult development has been termed sexist by some writers, his framework still provides some salient issues that both men and women deal with during various phases of the adult life cycle (Garner & Mercer, 1989; Goleman, 1990).

Although life-stage development theories provide a useful framework, they must be used with caution. These theories can be easily misused if they are interpreted to mean that all persons enter and exit each stage at a particular point in life. There is also a danger that people who are not grappling with the issues assigned to his or her age will be labeled developmentally delayed or "sick." We agree with Weick (1983) and Schlossberg (1984) that the assumption of "sequential growth" in adulthood needs to be challenged. Themes of adulthood do not necessarily emerge at only given moments of time, to be resolved and then forgotten. Rather, they are more cyclical in nature.

Every person charts a unique course through life, with various life events happening at unique times. Life-course development theory is based on the fact that many people experience certain life events (e.g. having children, death of parents, serious illnesses) at around the same age. As Rossi (1980) points out, however, these theories were developed at a time when people's lives were quite stable and uniform with respect to certain life events (e.g., marriage, having children) and that this is no longer the case. The theories are also based on studies of individuals in a particular culture (American), social class (middle upper), race (white), and gender (male). They should not be applied indiscriminately to other groups without further study.

Given these caveats, we do not use the data to prove any theory of life-course development, nor do we apply the theory indiscriminately to our population, which is comprised of women with a wider range of backgrounds than the populations on which the theories were based. Instead, we attempt to develop themes from the data, looking closely at the interviews of women in a particular life stage and only then examining developmental theories to see if there is an interaction. We have used the theory to expand on and further understand what women have told us about their experiences. The result is that for each chapter, some of the themes identified relate to life-course development theories, and some do not.

Experiencing Illness

A third tradition influencing this book comes from the field of medical sociology. Sociologists have been interested in illness since Parsons developed the notion of the "sick role" (Parsons, 1951), but only recently have they begun to consider illness from the viewpoint of the person who is ill rather than from the perspective of physicians and hospitals. In the introduction to their book on epilepsy, Schneider and Conrad (1983) review this literature, and argue that there is a need for "studies of the experience of illness (which are) grounded in systematically-collected, first-hand data and analyzed within a . . . social psychological framework" (pp. 14–15). The perspective of women with breast cancer has been largely ignored, despite a voluminous literature on the psychological aspects of breast cancer. As we did our interviews, we were more and more convinced that the voices of the women experiencing the illness needed to be heard. By presenting the experiences of women with breast cancer, we hope to make a contribution to the fledgling field of the sociology of illness experience.

Womens' Voices

A fourth tradition that has influenced us is the interest within the women's studies movement in creating a forum for women's voices. Gilligan (1982a, 1982b) and Miller (1986) have called for research that "would delineate in women's own terms the experience of their adult life" (Gilligan 1982a, p. 112). Gilligan and Miller have also stressed the importance of social relationships for women. In a more general sense, this book is affected by the recent thinking of scholars such as Belenky, Clinchy, Goldberger, and Tarule 1986) who suggest that the more traditional ways of gathering knowledge (e.g., the scientific method) have been shaped by a male-dominated culture that values highly the rational, logical approach. In the process, women's ways of knowing (based more on intuition, personal experience, and others' experience) have been hidden in a kind of underground.

In this book, we focus on the *experiences* of women with breast cancer. By relying on our own intuition and the connections we made with the women we interviewed, we also hope to contribute to the knowledge of the breast cancer experience in a different way than has been traditional in the field—a way that we think will be more meaningful to women. In this way the book will facilitate the kind of sharing of experience so important to women.

These four areas of knowledge—adaptation to illness, life-course development, experiencing illness, and women's voices—have been integrated into our book to provide a clearer understanding of the experiences and thoughts of women with breast cancer. The common set of tasks that we have selected as most appropriate to the experience of breast cancer and life-course development theory has been used to understand what issues are most focal for women's experiences with breast cancer at different life phases. The sociology of illness experience has influenced our work from the very beginning when we decided to understand breast cancer as an *experience* from the woman's viewpoint and to report the perceptions of how women cope with breast cancer. Feminist thinking informed our work both methodologically and substantively. Our methodology involved a case-study approach in which we did not label or quantify women's voices, but allowed these voices to speak more directly about actual experiences with breast cancer. Substantively, we have asked about and given a high priority to understanding the importance of social relationships for women, as a way that women learn and grow.

STUDY

Profile of Women Interviewed

Our goal was to learn about the experience of breast cancer from women representing the life stages of young, middle, and later adulthood. We interviewed only women who had had the diagnosis for at least one year so they would have had some time to gain perspective on their experience. We had no upper limit on time since diagnosis. We interviewed women from 1 to 21 years following initial diagnosis, although one half were interviewed within the first 3 years.

Our sample was one of convenience. We began by asking for volunteers at a lecture that was given at an American Cancer Society series. Snowballing techniques yielded another set of women, each of whom was approached by someone she knew, and, if she agreed, we were given information on how to contact her. When we had conducted about one half of the interviews, we reviewed the ages and characteristics of our sample and realized that it contained mostly women in their 30s, 40s, and 50s. We then began to seek out younger (20s) and older (60+) women, and women who had life-styles not thus far represented. We did this by contacting people who might know eligible women and letting them know the characteristics we were looking for. We contacted local chapters of the American Cancer Society, health professionals, breast cancer support group leaders, and a member of the lesbian community. We also made further announcements at the American Cancer Society lecture series and in a hospital women's health newsletter, specifically asking for older and younger women. Ultimately, we interviewed 42 women. In all cases, the women either volunteered or consented to have their name released to us. Required procedures were used to obtain informed consent and to obtain consent to tape the interviews. Confidentiality was assured for the participants.

The interviewees ranged in age at diagnosis from 26 to 79, with 17 women in young adulthood (under 40), 16 women in middle adulthood (40–59), and 9 women in later adulthood (60+). The women came mostly from Eastern seaboard cities, suburbs, and rural counties. A few came from the Midwest and Far West. Twenty-five were married, 10 were single, 4 were divorced, and 3 were widowed. Three women were black, and 2 were lesbians. We had a range of occupations including secretary, homemaker, bookkeeper, beautician, nun, nurse, social worker, accountant, realtor, teacher, administrator, lawyer, and scientist. Thirteen were homemakers, and we estimated that 15 were in service jobs and 14 were in professional jobs. They ranged from working class to upper class, with most falling into some type of middle class. Only the very lowest socioeconomic classes were not represented.

We estimated that 23 of the women had their cancer diagnosed when it was considered Stage I, 15 had Stage II cancer, and 2 were at more advanced stages at the time of diagnosis. (In 2 cases, we were unable to estimate the stage.) Eight of the women experienced recurrences since diagnosis, and 1 was waiting to find out if her cancer had recurred at the time of the interview. In terms of surgical treatments, 4 were originally treated with lumpectomy, 34 were originally treated with mastectomy, and 4 were originally treated with double mastectomy. At the time of the interview, 2 of the initial lumpectomy patients had had mastectomies, and 7 of the mastectomy patients had had a second mastectomy. Twelve of the women had had breast reconstruction. Twenty-two at some point had chemotherapy, 9 had radiation treatments, and 4 had hormonal treatments. These numbers indicate the number who had each treatment. They cannot be added because many women had multiple treatments.

Interviews

Because we wanted to capture the women's experiences, we did not want to overstructure the interviews. Instead, we asked each woman to tell us her story in her own words. Most women began with the medical history, and we probed how these experiences felt to her and what she thought at the time. We also asked how she felt the experience with breast cancer had affected her and how it might have affected her relationships with significant others. The interviews were more like conversations than structured interviews. The interviewer's role was to encourage the women to talk about their experience, to validate the importance of their ideas, and to provide support for their sharing. Most of the interviews lasted from 1 to 2 hours and were done in the homes of the women. All were tape-recorded and later transcribed. Thirty-five of the 42 interviews were done by the authors, 5 were completed by a doctoral student, and 2 were completed by a retired social worker. In one interview, a family member translated because the respondent did not speak English.

In one case, a respondent terminated the interview shortly after it began. She said she feared that talking about the effect of her breast cancer on her marriage would make her upset. With this one exception, the interviewing process went very smoothly. The women were generally very eager to talk with us and needed little prompting. Many said afterward that they had enjoyed the interview, and some said that they found it therapeutic.

Analysis

Qualitative research procedures were used to analyze the data. The goal was to review the transcripts within each life stage and to search for "emergent themes" (Glasser & Strauss, 1967). Transcripts were coded for life tasks, illness tasks, relationships, and other areas of importance to the interviewees (e.g., illness experiences). Themes were identified for each life stage, and were narrowed down to three or four that were particularly salient to the particular life stage. Sometimes, the same theme was identified in more than one stage, and we had to decide where to place it. In some cases, it was found on closer examination to fit better in one stage than another (e.g., marriage, discussed in all life stages, was most problematic for midlife women). Other issues, such as relationships with mothers, were felt to be relevant to more than one life stage and were discussed in both places. We began by selecting quotations to use in the analysis of the key themes. We were unhappy with the result, however, because the quotations were taken out of the context of the interview and were isolated from the individuals. Something vital was lost. We then decided to select several individuals from each life stage, looking for good illustrations of the themes and a variety of life-styles, and allow these women to tell their whole stories. These "case studies" were used in the analysis of the themes, and pertinent quotations from other women in each life stage were added. In preparing the final manuscript, at least one observation or quotation was used from each of the 42 interviews we conducted.

Considerable editorial license was used to create the case studies from the transcripts. First names, locations, and occupations were changed to protect the confidentiality of the women. We also omitted information on race and sexual orientation for the same reason. Because the sample was small, generalizations about differences based on these characteristics would be inappropriate. If ideas about how these characteristics affect the breast cancer experience were made by the women themselves, however, they were included.

The order of quotations was changed, and material considered tangential was omitted. In addition, the spoken language was altered in minor ways to be understandable in written language. That is, expressions like "you know" were omitted, incomplete sentences were completed, tenses were changed, and so forth. In all cases, our goal in making these editorial changes was to better communicate what the respondent was saying. Because this type of editing can accidentally change the meaning, all case studies were returned to the women on whose transcripts they were based, and they were asked to let us know if we had misinterpreted anything they wanted to say. Almost all requested that some changes be made, but the changes requested were largely cosmetic, and little was challenged because of misinterpretation. Several respondents wanted us to change negative comments they had made about relatives. We complied with all these requests, although we thought they made the book a little less colorful

Because there were two authors involved, it is important to add that this analysis involved a process in which we worked both independently and together. We shared our initial impressions, our ideas as they emerged, our feelings and thoughts about each interview, and our written work. We each interviewed people of all ages, but Carolyn initially drafted the chapters on young adulthood (20s) and middle adulthood, and Julianne drafted the chapter on breast cancer and its treatment, and the chapters on young adulthood (30s) and later adulthood. We then exchanged drafts and added, deleted, and commented on each other's work. Through this process our ideas became clarified and focused. We were then tempted to write much too much—to include every relevant quote and every interesting thought. Much has been left (painfully) on the cutting room floor. We hope that the result communicates our ideas clearly, without being too concise. The two authors contributed equally to the final manuscript, the order of our names reflecting only the alphabet.

Limitations

Because we did not select a random sample, and because the sample is small, it would be a mistake to try to generalize our findings to all women with breast cancer. By relying on volunteers, we probably excluded women who were not comfortable talking about their cancer experiences. We also found women through community-based programs, so that we have a large number of women who are active in these programs. This research is cross-sectional, rather than longitudinal, and brings with it the limits of examining a person's experience at only one point in time.

Another problem was created by the wide range in the length of time that had elapsed between time of diagnosis and time of interview. Those who were fairly close to the diagnosis were likely to be in the same life stage at the interview as at the diagnosis. Twelve women, however, were interviewed in a different life stage at the interview than they were at diagnosis. We realized that the perspective of these women could have been influenced by this, and had to decide whether to count them by the diagnosis or the interview. We decided to consider them to be in the life stage they were at time of diagnosis, because we were focusing primarily on events following the diagnosis. There was one exception to this pattern. One woman was 58 at diagnosis and had a metastasis at 71. We interviewed her after the cancer had metastasized and counted her in the later stage of adulthood.

It is also important to remember that all of the information reported on the sample came from interviews with the women themselves. We did not review medical records, nor did we speak with family members or others who may have had information on the woman and how she reacted. This is appropriate because we were focusing on how the women experienced the breast cancer, but it means that all the information is subjective. Finally, although we made special efforts to locate older women, this population is underrepresented in our sample, because breast cancer is most prevalent in this age group. In chapter 6, the analysis suggests some reasons why this group may not have been easily accessible to us.

In keeping with the nature of the sample, we do not try to quantify the results or use them to test hypotheses. Instead, we rely on quotations and case studies to present these women's experiences.

OVERVIEW

Chapter 1 reviews basic information about breast cancer and its treatment. This information is presented to help the reader understand the experiences described in the case studies in the later chapters of the book. It covers the literature about the impact of breast cancer on women and explores women's experiences and reactions. The major illness tasks faced by a breast cancer patient are delineated. These tasks include (a) handling some of the major psychological reactions (denial, anger, anxiety, and self-absorption); (b) preserving a satisfactory body image; (c) maintaining satisfying sexual relationships; (d) adjusting to role shifts; and (e) dealing with an uncertain future. Also discussed in this chapter is the importance to these women of social relationships and social support. Finally, the literature on age and adjustment to breast cancer is discussed.

In chapters 2 and 3 the issues of breast cancer in the young adult are discussed. In chapter 2, the focus is on young women in the first phase of young adulthood (the 20s). Case histories presented are (a) Rosemary, age 26, a single woman who worked in an insurance agency; (b) Karen, age 28, a single woman who was a speech therapist attending graduate school at night; and (c) Ingrid, age 28, a married health educator whose cancer had metastasized and who was living at home with her parents. The themes that surfaced as particularly important for women in their 20s with breast cancer were "achieving independence," "fertility," "developing intimate relationships," and "finding a place in the adult world."

Chapter 3 begins with the stories of (a) Dorothy, age 34, a physician, married with two children; (b) Ruth, age 36, a psychiatric nurse, who was married with two small children; and (c) Laura, age 38, a single woman who was a scientist working in a government laboratory. The themes that were salient for women in their 30s—"letting go of the just world idea," "sexuality," "coping with children," "relationships with mothers," and "evaluating the meaning of work"—are addressed as they intersect with breast cancer tasks.

Chapters 4 and 5 are devoted to midlife women (40–59). Two chapters were needed for this phase because there was simply too much material for one chapter. Unfortunately, however, there was no clear-cut way to divide the material. It could not be divided easily into two distinct phases, as was possible in young adulthood. Therefore, the division is arbitrary, and was made by dividing the themes and then using case studies that best illustrate these themes. In chapter 4 we address three issues important to midlife women: "body image," "marriage," and "relationships with adolescent children." The cases of (a) Jessica, age 45, in her second marriage who has a teenage son; (b) Beth, diagnosed at age 51, married with five children and working part-time; and (c) Sandra, age 40, a suburban homemaker and part-time student who had four children, are presented to illustrate the concerns of married midlife women with breast cancer.

In chapter 5, additional themes that were prevalent in our interviews with midlife women who have breast cancer are discussed. The lives of three women, (a) Diane, age 46, an administrator; (b) Wanda, age 48, a retired travel agent; and (c) Gwen, age 59, a teacher, are presented to illuminate the midlife themes of "confronting death," "reassessing one's life," "self-reliance," "generativity," "relationships with mothers," and "friendships."

The lives of four women in later adulthood are presented in chapter 6: (a) Emily, age 69 at diagnosis, an active community volunteer, married with adult children and grandchildren; (b) Judith, single all her life, diagnosed at age 63 after early retirement from her job with a major corporation; (c) Linda, a 66-year-old widow, with several grandchildren; and (d) Elizabeth, whose breast cancer recurred at age 71, who had once owned a successful business. Themes common to the experiences of older women diagnosed with breast cancer—"coping with losses," "relationships with children," "independence," and "depression-despair"—are discussed.

The major goal of the book is to explore the intersection of breast cancer tasks and life-course development. This book also provides an opportunity for women with breast cancer to share their experiences with other women coping with this disease. The following quote from a book of poems written by breast cancer patients (Lifshitz, 1988) summarizes an important goal of our book.

> Silence encourages denial, trivialization, and ignorance. It helps no one—not the person who needs to share or the person who needs to know. Women have always shared. It has been a way to make vital connections and a way to survive. (p. xviii).

Other goals include understanding illness as it is experienced and helping health professionals to better serve the needs of women with breast cancer. Although this book is based on breast cancer, the model developed may be applicable to other illnesses in women as well. It would not be appropriate to transfer this model to all such illness experiences, but we hope that further research will explore its applicability. We envision the audience for this book to be health care professionals such as social workers, psychologists, counselors, psychiatrists, nurses and physicians, and women who have breast cancer as well as their family members and friends.

1 The Experience of Breast Cancer and Its Treatments

Although this book deals with breast cancer in the life course, we begin with a description of the basic medical and psychosocial aspects of breast cancer and its treatments that are common to women of all ages. This material is included to provide the information needed to understand the case studies presented in subsequent chapters. It is not a complete or definitive discussion of breast cancer, and it is not intended for use as a guide to treatment decisions. In chapters 2 to 6, we consider how these common experiences impact on women at different points in their lives. It is our thesis that although all women with breast cancer have a set of common experiences and "tasks," where they are in the life course will affect which aspects of these common experiences are most salient to them.

We begin with a brief description of the disease of breast cancer, and then cover the steps a woman goes through as breast cancer is diagnosed and treated. The medical information in this chapter, unless cited otherwise, comes from the *Breast Cancer Digest* (National Cancer Institute, 1984). We include quotations from women in our sample to describe how each of these steps is experienced. We then discuss the socioemotional "tasks" that are common to all women with breast cancer, illustrating these with quotations from women in our sample. Also included is a discussion of social support and the importance of social relationships for women. Finally, the chapter argues that age and adaptation to breast cancer have not been adequately studied in relation to social relationships and socioemotional illness tasks.

MEDICAL ASPECTS OF BREAST CANCER AND ITS TREATMENT

Breast cancer is the commonest form of cancer among American women, with 1 in 10 women affected at some point in her life. It is also the second most frequent cause of cancer death in women, only recently surpassed by lung cancer. The incidence of breast cancer is closely associated with age, with rates of about 1 in 100,000 for those 20 to 25 years old, rising to about 100 in 100,000 for those 40 to 44, and about 300 in 100,000 for those aged 70 to 74 years.

All cancer involves cells that are characterized by uncontrolled growth. Breast cancers are categorized in several ways: First, they are categorized as carcinomas (99%) (which arise in the breast tissue) or sarcomas (1%) (which arise in the connective tissue or support structure of the breast). Another categorization is ductal cancer (89%) (arises in the breast ducts, which carry milk to the nipple) or lobular cancer (5%) (arises in the lobes, where milk is produced); Paget's disease (3%) and inflammatory carcinoma (3%) account for the rest. Finally, breast cancers can be invasive (94%) (have broken through the borders of the ducts and invaded surrounding tissue) or noninvasive, also called in situ (6%), (confined to the ducts or lobes). About 70% of the cases of breast cancer are invasive ductal at the time of diagnosis.

Breast cancers vary widely in rate of growth. Some double their size (diameter) in only a few days, and others take more than a year to double. By the time a slow-growing cancer in the breast is big enough to be felt, it may have been in the breast for years. Breast cancers also vary with respect to size, contour (smooth or irregular), type of cells (e.g., poorly differentiated), and location. About 50% of breast cancers occur in the upper, outer quadrant of the breast. Cancers that are closer to the lymph nodes are thought to spread faster. Another factor that differs about breast cancers is whether they respond to the female hormones estrogen and progesterone. If so, these hormones can be used to control the growth of the cancer.

Breast cancers spread to other parts of the body through the lymphatic system and the blood vessels. When breast cancers spread (metastasize), the lymph nodes are usually affected. For this reason, lymph nodes in the underarm (axilla) are usually removed and examined once a breast cancer has been found, to see if the cancer has the ability to spread. This information helps determine prognosis and treatment. If there are positive lymph nodes, the prognosis is not as good.

Detection and Diagnosis

There were two major routes to the discovery of breast cancer in our study. Some women had a mammogram (breast x-ray) that detected a cancer. Others had found a sign, such as a lump or discharge from a nipple. Almost all of the women we talked with were initially reassured by their physicians that there was no need to worry. Although this initial reassurance is undoubtedly because most breast lumps are benign (80% of those biopsied are not cancer), it left many women in our study with a lack of confidence when reassurance was provided later by the doctor.

Women who are diagnosed by mammogram may have a difficult time believing that they really have cancer. For one 60-year-old woman, her first mammogram turned up as cancer. She questioned why she had to go through such aggressive treatment (mastectomy and chemotherapy) when she had never even felt sick.

Although one may imagine that finding a lump would be very frightening for women, most of the women we talked with also felt some uncertainty. One woman waited for weeks after finding a lump, and then had her husband and daughter feel the lump before she called her doctor. It is often difficult for women to tell if what they feel is really a lump. One half of all women have lumpy breasts, and most of these lumps are not cancerous. So, when a woman reports feeling a lump to her doctor, she is usually told that it is probably nothing. In premenopausal women, these lumps are affected by the hormones that regulate menstruation. These women are often told to watch the lump for a while and to see if it goes down after her period. If this has happened, perhaps several times, the woman learns to think twice about reporting it. It was not uncommon for the women in our sample to have had previous lumps. In this case, the discovery of a new lump brought on a variety of emotions: fear, of course, that this time it might be cancer but also annoyance—that another biopsy would need to be done only to find another benign lump. "Do you go through life removing one lump every 2 years? I'm sick of all these lumps!" complains one woman. Like the boy who cried "wolf," she never knows if the next one will be cancerous. A lump is not the only sign of breast cancer, however. One woman experienced bleeding from her nipple, but did not recognize this as a sign of breast cancer (see case study on Jessica in chapter 4).

Once a breast lump is discovered, either by mammogram or palpation (feeling it), an evaluation is necessary to determine whether it is cancerous or not. This is usually done with a combination of mammography and biopsy. There are two common types of biopsy: needle biopsies and surgical biopsies. Needle biopsies, which can be fine needle (aspiration), which removes fluid, or wide needle, which removes tissue, are done in the physician's office, under local anesthetic. If the lump is benign, fluid can often be extracted, and the lump disappears. When fluid cannot be withdrawn, the mass remains, or examination of the fluid shows cancer cells, a solid (cancerous) tumor is suspected, and a surgical biopsy is recommended. There are two types of surgical biopsies: excisional and incisional. In the excisional surgical biopsy, the entire mass is removed and sent to pathology to be analyzed. In the incisional biopsy, usually done on larger tumors, a sample of the lump is removed and examined. When a biopsy is done on a lump that is not palpable (e.g., one that cannot be felt and is seen only on mammogram), the surgeon must use special techniques to locate the tissue to be removed. Although most of the women in our study were concerned at this point with the *results* of the biopsy and not the biopsy itself, some women who had this type of biopsy found it very uncomfortable. One woman (see case study on Linda in chapter 6) reports the following.

> He took this long, skinny wire and started inserting it into the breast. They don't give you anything [anesthesia]. And they push it down and push. And I think, "Am I really sitting here going through this? This is the worst thing I've ever had in my life!"

Another woman (age 79) was more concerned about the way she was treated than with the pain.

> After about 12 x-rays, she began—she had some—oh, it looked like a crochet hook. She hooked that into my skin. It wasn't terribly painful. Just very uncomfortable. Then, they made me get up and *walk* down the hall to the surgery. I did not have anything on above me. She gave me a towel, but it wasn't a long one. It was embarrassing. I felt that she belittled me.

After the tissue is removed, it can be examined in two ways: by frozen section (which takes about 30 min) or by permanent section (which takes 24 hr but is more accurate). Until recently, frozen sections were used because the biopsy and mastectomy were performed in the same operation. If the frozen section was positive, a mastectomy was performed immediately. Since the late 1970s, owing in large part to the influence of Kushner (1975), this is less and less common. Today, a two-step procedure, using a permanent section, is standard and is even mandated in several states. This has several advantages. Its results are more accurate, and it provides women some time to consider treatment options, to get second opinions, have tests to see if the cancer has spread, to explore the option of reconstruction, and to get ready psychologically for treatment.

If a biopsy is positive, several tests are done to determine the stage of the disease and the prognosis. The lower the stage, the better the prognosis. In situ tumors are considered precancerous. Stage I cancers are small (< 2 cm) and no affected lymph nodes are found. When the tumor is larger (between 2 and 5 cm) or lymph nodes are positive, then the cancer is classified as Stage II. Stage III involves a larger tumor (> 5 cm) or spread to contiguous areas. If there is evidence of spread to distant areas (metastases), the cancer is called Stage IV. Five-year survival rates vary considerably with stage of disease. For example, 85% of white women with Stage I disease are alive 5 years after the diagnosis, compared to only 10% of those with Stage IV disease.

Other factors (beyond tumor size and spread) that influence prognosis include the nature of the tumor (whether it is slow or fast growing, where it is located, whether it responds to the hormones estrogen and progesterone); the strength of the immune system, the patient's age (breast cancers in younger women are usually more aggressive); and weight and reproductive history.

Getting the News

Learning the results of the biopsy is often the time when women experience the most intense anxiety. Waiting for the results of tests can be agonizing. Anything that can be done to get the results to women quickly would be highly desirable.

In almost all cases, the women in our study knew that the results of the biopsy were positive before actually being told. They sensed the results from the physician's tone of voice or facial expression. One woman reports, "He [the surgeon] asked if I had come in alone. As soon as he said that, I knew." Nancy (age 36) puts it this way, "I could tell by his initial disappointment when he came into the recovery room."

One problem is that at the point of finding out that she has cancer, a woman's anxiety skyrockets. At this time, it is very difficult for her to absorb any new information. Doctors often use this time to review treatment options, however, and to generally educate women about breast cancer. Not surprisingly, women often do not retain this information. Sylvia (age 56) relates her experience this way.

> When I sat down at his desk, he said, "You have breast cancer." And the adrenalin started BOOM-BOOM-BOOM BOOM-BOOM-BOOM! To be perfectly honest, he threw medical terminology at me that—it was Greek! I didn't know what he was saying. I was petrified! So he said, "Here are your options," and blah blah blah. And I said, "Excuse me, doctor. Could you stop for a minute?" I said, "To you, cancer is an everyday word. To me, it's a frightening word. I'm not hearing you."

It is perhaps in part because of this that women widely report not having been informed about what to expect from treatment for breast cancer (Hailey, Lavine, & Hogan, 1988; Lindsey, Norbeck, Carrieri, & Perry, 1981).

Selection of Physicians

One factor that occupies many women in the period before treatment begins is the choice of physicians. Some women stay with the doctor they saw originally for discovery of the lump, who is often a general practitioner or a gynecologist. Most select a surgeon for the biopsy and any surgical treatment, and many also select an oncologist. Some will also need a radiotherapist and a plastic surgeon for reconstruction. The women in our study had very different experiences in selecting and interacting with doctors. It must be remembered that women are required to make a very important set of decisions at a time when they are feeling highly anxious and vulnerable. Some women simply take the easiest path, accepting the referral of their primary care physician. Others take a more active role in their own health care, finding that selecting a physician provides a sense of control at a time when life seems to have gone out of control.

One woman reports the following.

> Finding the right oncologist is very important. We went down to the [University Cancer Center], and the doctors down there said I would get the standard chemotherapy treatment—nothing experimental. The Cancer Center is like a zoo. My husband said it looked like a bunch of drug addicts waiting for their fix! He was hoping that I wouldn't have to go there. So I chose the local county hospital. And I chose a doctor who was young and good looking. I thought that was important, since he was going to bother me every two weeks!

Another factor she mentioned was the doctor's approach to treatment. "He was very conservative and didn't want to take any chances. I didn't want an oncologist who was going to say, 'Oh, you're having nausea or you're having this or that [side effect] so I'll go easy on you [lower the dosage].' I wanted someone who would push me to where it is effective. And he did. He ended up giving me twice the dosage the doctor at [the cancer center] recommended!"

Sylvia (age 56) had seen two surgeons, and selected the one who proposed a shorter course of radiation. "That didn't determine it; I could have gone through the 2 weeks more, but it was just that he was stoic, and I didn't like his personality. He wasn't going to be able to help me emotionally." Roberta (age 31) rejected a doctor for being too depressing.

> One doctor that I talked with, every time I'd see him or talk to him, everything was so serious and just so depressing. He was always saying things like "I'm so sorry you have to go through this!" The other doctors were not like that. I would come out of his office in tears all the time, and I thought, "This is ridiculous! I don't have to subject myself to that!" I finally decided not to see him anymore.

These comments suggest that socioemotional factors are important to women selecting doctors. Also, women look for a doctor who provides support for their coping style. For each of the three women mentioned earlier, there was another woman in our sample who made the exact opposite decision. Elizabeth (chapter 6) switched to a cancer center after trying a local doctor and finding she was not getting enough information. A woman who is a stoic herself (e.g., see Jeanne in chapter 6) might have liked the doctor Sylvia rejected. Ruth (chapter 3), who worked through her depression very openly, might have appreciated the doctor Roberta found too depressing.

Finally, just having the opportunity to make a choice is probably helpful to women. Wanda (chapter 5) is an example of a woman who did not, and who to this day blames her radical mastectomy on the fact that she did not have a good relationship with her surgeon.

Choosing Treatment

Only recently, the major treatment for breast cancer was a radical mastectomy, in which the breast was removed surgically, along with the underarm lymph nodes and the chest muscles. This procedure leaves a hollow in the chest area. Research in the 1970s showed that a less radical procedure—called the modified radical mastectomy—was equally successful in treating breast cancer. This procedure removes the breast, the underarm lymph nodes, and the lining over the chest muscle. The operation is less deforming because the chest muscle is left intact. Now, research is showing equally good results with an even *less* radical procedure—lumpectomy—when it is combined with radiation (Fisher, Redmond, Fisher, 1985; Fisher, Redmond, Poisson, 1989). In this procedure, only the breast lump is removed. Some of the underarm lymph nodes are also usually removed to test for any spread of the cancer. The remainder of the breast is usually treated with radiation (see discussion of radiation later in this chapter.) A National Institutes of Health panel recommended lumpectomy with radiation for early breast cancer in 1990 on the grounds that long-term survival is the same, and the breast is preserved. A woman who undergoes lumpectomy without radiation has an increased risk for a recurrence in the breast; however, with treatment, she has the same chance of disease-free, long-term survival as does the woman who has a mastectomy (A. Dorr, personal communication, 1990).

Women with early-stage breast cancer now often have a choice between modified radical mastectomy and lumpectomy with or without radiation. Because lumpectomies have been offered as an alternative for some women, there has been a spate of research comparing the psychological outcome of the two operations. Most of this research has shown no difference in levels of anxiety or depression, the most often measured variables (Baider, Rizel, & DeNour, 1986; Fallowfield, Baum, & Maguire,

1987; Holmberg, Omne-Ponten, Burns, Adami, & Bergstrom, 1989; Meyer & Aspergren, 1989; Sanger & Reznikoff, 1981; Steinberg, Juliano, and Wise 1985; Wolberg, Romsaas, Tanner, & Malec, 1989). Some literature has suggested, however, that women receiving lumpectomies have better outcomes in areas related to body image, body satisfaction, sexual enjoyment, and feelings of attractiveness (Kemeney, Wellisch, & Schain, 1988; Margolis, Goodman, & Rubin, 1990; Meyer & Aspergren, 1989; Sanger & Reznikoff, 1981; Steinberg et al., 1985). In evaluating these studies, it is important to remember that some involve women who were randomly assigned to treatment. Although this may be the best way to determine that any differences in outcomes found are due to the treatments and not to preexisting differences, it does not reflect the situation of a woman who is involved in choosing one treatment over another.

Having a choice of treatment can have both positive and negative effects. On the positive side, there is evidence that women who are given a choice have better outcomes than those who are not, regardless of the treatment chosen (Dean, 1988; Maguire, 1989; Morris, 1988; Morris & Ingham, 1988; Morris & Royle, 1988). Conversely, for some women, the element of choice increases anxiety. According to Holland and Mastrovito (1980), "Increasing patient responsibility in treatment increases the number of decisions the patient must make, and this has, at times, led to increased anxiety about contemplating alternative approaches to treatment" (p. 1046). Holland and Rowland (1987) identify four different response types. Type I ("You decide for me, doctor") is most often an older woman. Type II ("I demand you do the _____ procedure") is common among young women who are well read. Type III ("I can't decide") is seen in women who are overwhelmed by the situation. Type IV, which the authors feel represents the mature woman, responds: "Given the options, your recommendations, and my preferences, I choose _____." Again, one problem is that at the time women have to make this decision, they are highly anxious and, as a result, their reasoning and concentration are lower than normal (Holland & Rowland, 1987).

In our study, we found that different women approached this choice in different ways. One woman describes her decision in the following way.

> "Now," he said "there are options—lumpectomy and then radiation." Well, I didn't like the idea of going through radiation if I didn't have to. And you really have no choice. You really don't. I mean, you're dealing with cancer, not a cold or a broken foot. And you don't fool around with cancer. You're asking for a cure, and you go for as sure a treatment as you can.

She chose mastectomy, but, between her biopsy and the surgery, she found some pressure to reconsider.

What started happening is, these "experts" started coming out of the wood-
work. People who have never had breast cancer are telling you all kinds of
information about what they heard, whose friend did this and why don't you
do that? People come up to you and say, "Why don't you have a lumpectomy?" "Why don't you go for a second opinion?" It's like people planting
seeds of doubt. It's almost like they're calling you a fool because you're
choosing [the mastectomy]. It was insane!

Another woman we interviewed had a similar experience, with a
different outcome. When her doctor said she was a "perfect candidate" for
lumpectomy, she worried that she would be a guinea pig. She also objected
to radiation, because her brother had had a bad experience with it. When
she decided to have a mastectomy, however, her daughters thought she
was crazy and talked her into the lumpectomy. She went through lumpectomy and radiation, and is pleased with the cosmetic result, but she says
that if she gets cancer again, she "wouldn't play Russian roulette. It
wouldn't be lumpectomy again—it would be mastectomy."

Although research shows that the survival rates of mastectomy and
lumpectomy-radiation patients are equal, it seems that these women
viewed lumpectomy as more risky. They seemed to feel that the choice
they are given is not two equally effective treatments, but a choice between
their looks and their lives. In fact, Holland and Rowland (1987) report that
"observations from our clinical practice indicate elevated fears of recurrence among patients undergoing combined lumpectomy-irradiation"
(p. 641). Although there is evidence that having a choice can be beneficial, it also leaves women in a position of having to defend their choice
to others. If they chose lumpectomy, they may feel that they are "vain,"
and that they will always have to worry (and feel guilty) about recurrence. If they chose mastectomy, they are criticized for being "foolish,"
sacrificing a breast unnecessarily. Nor is a choice necessarily permanent.
One woman did extensive research, and opted for lumpectomy. After the
lumpectomy, however, the tissue was examined and a very virulent form
of cancer was found. Because recurrence was common with this type of
cancer, and spread was very rapid, she ended up with bilateral mastectomies.

One concern we heard about the decision was that some women felt
they did not have adequate time to make it. One woman complained,
"They give you so little time. They give you the weekend!" One wonders if
some women are being rushed into decisions they may later come to
regret. It is also possible that when the time a woman is given to make a
decision is limited, more mastectomies are chosen then would otherwise
be the case. Under great anxiety, with limited time to calm down and sort
things out, many women may opt for the "safest" and least controversial
option.

There is some evidence that women who are more concerned with body image choose lumpectomy-radiation, whereas those who have a greater fear of death tend to choose mastectomy (Margolis, Goodman, Rubin, & Pajac, 1989; Wolberg, Tanner, Romsaas, Trump, & Malec, 1987). If these findings hold up in further studies, it may be possible to develop inventories that women could use to rate the importance of different factors to them. Although many physicians seem comfortable recommending one option or the other based on *physical* criteria (e.g., size of breast, size of lump, age), they might also do well to consider psychological variations.

One factor that many of the women found important, but that was not usually considered in the treatment decision, was sensation. For many women, the breast is an important erogenous zone. The loss of this threatens a loss of sexual responsiveness and pleasure. Although heavy attention is paid to how the breast *looks* (the partner's perspective) the question of how it will *feel* (the woman's perspective) is often ignored. Physicians who recommend mastectomy with reconstruction may be minimizing the importance of the fact that the reconstructed breast has no feeling. Women who choose lumpectomy-radiation may be unaware of the possibility of changes in sensation in the skin, including either reduced or increased sensation. The breast often feels firmer, and in some cases the size changes as well. In the mastectomy or lumpectomy-radiation decision, one factor that should be added is the importance to the individual woman of the breast in her sexual responses, and the impact that the various choices may have on this.

Finally, there is presently a difference in the type of supportive services available for the two surgical operations. The American Cancer Society has developed several programs to support women with breast cancer (e.g., Reach to Recovery), and there are support groups in hospitals throughout the country; however, these programs tend to be dominated by women who have had mastectomies. When support groups are open to women with lumpectomies, but not exclusively for them, they may feel unwelcome. One woman who had a lumpectomy relates the following experience.

> I joined the breast group at ——— Hospital, but I stopped going. It was all mastectomy. When I mentioned that I had had a lumpectomy, a couple of women looked at me—and not being paranoid or anything, I thought they were thinking "What is she doing here?" I asked around, and I was the only lumpectomy. I felt kind of bad for them that here I had my breast, and they didn't.

This experience suggests that the woman with a lumpectomy may be cut off from some of the traditional support available for women with mastectomies. Perhaps as more women have lumpectomies, and as more recognition is given to the fact that adjusting to breast cancer involves more than just adjusting to the loss of a breast, services will be developed to provide support for this population.

Before leaving the topic of choosing treatment, it is important to point out that some women may want to consider not having any surgical treatment. If the cancer has metatasized, it may be too late for surgery on the breast to do any good. If the cancer is not likely to spread (e.g., an extremely slow-growing type), surgery may not be necessary.

Surgery

Whether a mastectomy or a lumpectomy is done, most women with breast cancer are treated with surgery. Most receive mastectomies, although the frequency of lumpectomy is increasing.

Mastectomy

In our sample, 19 women (45%) were treated with mastectomy alone. In general, these women had early (Stage I) cancers, and they were able to return to normal activities fairly soon. Other women had mastectomy, or double mastectomy, combined with other (adjuvant) therapies.

Once a decision for mastectomy is made, a decision will be made about when to schedule the surgery. Some women in our sample were very eager to get the surgery over with. One woman puts it this way. "I took a tub bath because I knew that bathing would be difficult for a while, and when I looked down at my breast, I wanted it gone." Another woman bargained with her physician to postpone her surgery until after she had completed several activities she was already committed to. She scheduled the surgery 4 weeks after the biopsy. In retrospect, she feels that 4 weeks was too much time. "It gets to the point where you say 'Let's just get this over with!' "

Recovery from the surgery is usually rapid, although some pain around the wound, or "phantom" pain in the removed breast, is not unusual. Some type of drain is usually inserted to remove fluid from under the skin. Stitches and drains are removed within 1 to 2 weeks of the surgery. Women in our sample who had experienced other types of surgery in the past emphasized that a mastectomy is not nearly as traumatic medically as it is psychologically. No internal organs are involved; the wound is external. It is usually only when the bandages are removed that the reality of the surgery hits them.

One woman, who had a radical mastectomy, told us that it took her 2 years to look at the scar (see case study on Wanda in chapter 5). Another woman, who had bilateral (modified radical) mastectomies expected to have a similar reaction.

> I had thought that I would never show him [the husband], that I would go in the bathroom and get dressed. But I showed him in only a day or two. I do not think he wanted to see. I think I wanted him to say, "That doesn't look bad at all. It looks a lot better than I thought it would look!" But I could tell from his face that he wasn't thinking that [laughs]. But no wonder! I mean, I was all stitched, and it was a mess! It probably scared him to death. But it was just really important for me to show him at that moment, for some reason, and after that things were fine.

Northouse (1989) reports that in fact most husbands reacted well to seeing the mastectomy scar, but that a small group reported that it was a difficult experience.

A woman with three teenagers describes her return home from the hospital.

> I wasn't in this door five minutes that everybody wanted to see my scar. They said, "Well, let's see, let's see!" Of course, 23 staples stapled across my chest. "Let's see, let's see." And I had to show them. I had read about other women's reactions, "Oh, I couldn't look in the mirror for months!" But that's not how I felt. Because it's just a breast. It's not that important. It's not an arm or a leg or your sight . . . just fatty tissue. It didn't make me any less of a person than I am.

PROSTHESES   Most of the women in our study who had mastectomies were given a temporary prosthesis while in the hospital by a Reach to Recovery volunteer. Unless immediate reconstruction is done, women can purchase prostheses that duplicate their individual size and shape. Prostheses come in a large variety of materials, which differ in weight and texture. Some come with nipples. Most women in our study were very pleased with the way their prostheses looked, although they were not always satisfied with how they felt.

> I use a prosthesis, and I perspire a lot, especially in the summer. The prosthesis gets a mustylike smell. It stays wet all of the time. Most of the time [the prosthesis] is OK. I haven't had any problem about clothes. I don't wear any low-cut things. And anything sleeveless would show the cuts under my arms, so I try to get tops with a little sleeve. But when I was visiting my mother's home at Christmas, I was ready to leave, and I said, "I can't find my boobs." So everybody was looking for them. My sister was worried that her children would get ahold of them.
>
> Clara, age 52

I swam 2 weeks after the operation [mastectomy], but I had to get a prothesis for the bathing suit. And if you don't think that's a pain! When I'd stoop to get out of the pool, the suit would fall away from me on one side, and here I am, down to here [gestures to her waist]! It would be so obvious!

I have three different prostheses, because the silicon one is too heavy for running. It bounces. Even my natural self didn't bounce like that! The one I use for swimming gives you the shape, but it is light and doesn't bounce.

Marian, age 56

One elderly woman refused to wear her prosthesis. "I couldn't even wear it. It weighed a ton! I gave it up. I wanted my own bra. I put a little cotton padding in [my bra]. The other weighed a ton. My shoulder hurt from it, believe me."

Lumpectomy

Lumpectomy is essentially the same as a surgical biopsy except that a margin of surrounding tissue is also removed. Lumpectomy is usually combined with radiation therapy. The surgery leaves a scar, and, depending on the size of the excision relative to the size of the breast, some disfigurement of the breast can result. The side effects from the lymph node removal, and from the radiation, are generally severer than the lumpectomy itself. In our sample, 14% of the women had lumpectomies. Sylvia (age 56) describes the result of her lumpectomy as follows: "My breast doesn't look any different than when I went in to have my surgery, except that I have about that much of a scar, and there's a small indentation there."

Axillary Node Surgery

Whether a woman has lumpectomy or mastectomy, a sample of lymph nodes is usually removed to help decide if additional treatment is needed. One possible complication of this surgery is lymphedema, or swelling of the arm. This occurs when lymph and blood vessels are cut during the surgery and excess lymph fluid accumulates in the woman's arm. This is a common occurrence, but is severe in only about 10% of women. Only one of the women in our study had a serious problem with this symptom. Sylvia, who was so pleased with the results of her lumpectomy, was not happy with the scar from the removal of her lymph nodes ("I have quite a hole there"). Jeanne (age 72) also had scarring from the removal of her lymph nodes. "I have so much scar tissue, all up here [gestures] and all the way down. I had a lot of problems moving. It was the strain and the pull in the armpit. I still feel the discomfort of it. I can *do* everything, but I can't wear anything sleeveless." It may be that women who have mastectomies expect to have scarring and a period of recuperation, whereas those who have lumpectomies do not. Perhaps these women need to be better prepared for the effects of the removal of the lymph nodes, especially if they selected lumpectomy thinking that there would be *no* visible deformity.

Another common complication is arm and shoulder stiffness. Most women in our study were able to use exercises to reduce this and return to normal activities fairly quickly.

Radiation

As previously mentioned, women who chose lumpectomy usually have radiation treatment to the remaining part of the breast. Radiation is also sometimes used as primary treatment and to shrink large tumors in locally advanced disease. Following the surgery, women come in to a radiation treatment center for a series of external radiation treatments. The treatments take only a few minutes, and must be repeated 4 to 5 times a week for 4 or 5 consecutive weeks. To know where to focus the radiation beams, radiologists circle the area to be treated with small tattooed dots. These dots cannot be removed. The radiation series is usually followed by a "boost" of radiation to the tumor site. This may be done with an electron beam, which requires another 5 to 10 days of outpatient treatment, or with an implant (where irradiated tubes are implanted into the breast tissue for about 3 days). The implant requires a hospital stay.

Side effects of radiation can be fatigue, changes to the skin, such as sunburn or enlarged pores, changes in sensation (either increase or decrease), a firming of the breast tissue, and lymphedema. Some women experience a change in the size of the breast, and some report long-term soreness in the chest wall. When radiation gets into the lung, shortness of breath or coughing may result. In rare cases, ribs beneath the breast are weakened and may fracture. There is some evidence that women experiencing radiation therapy have psychological difficulty during the period of treatment (Hughson, Cooper, McArdle, & Smith, 1987; Meyerowitz, 1980; Silberfarb, Maurer, & Crouthamel, 1980), and that some become anxious around the time the treatment ends (Holland, Rowland, Lebovits, & Rusalem, 1979). In our sample, several women experienced panic attacks during radiation treatment or preparation for treatment.

Some women in our study decided not to have the breast-conserving surgery because they wanted to avoid radiation. Many were very afraid of any exposure to radiation, in some cases because friends or family members had had bad experiences in the past. Some could not manage radiation because the treatment schedule could not be fitted into their busy life-styles. Also, transportation to a radiation treatment center was not available to some women. This could be because they lived too far away, or because they did not drive and did not want to inconvenience others with such a burdensome schedule.

One woman, who had both chemotherapy and radiation reported, "I liked the radiation a whole lot better [than chemotherapy] because it didn't show. You know, chemotherapy showed. And I could get on a train and go to the hospital every day, just like I had a job for 6 weeks. So I kind of liked that."

Another woman, 70 at the time of her diagnosis, had bilateral mastectomies. She was adamantly opposed to any chemotherapy but agreed to a course of radiation therapy.

> I was going into my 4th week, and I thought, "Gee! I'm really lucky. My blood count is fine; I haven't lost my appetite; I was never nauseated, and I didn't have any burns." Suddenly, guess what? They're tacking eight more booster treatments onto me! After that, it all began to pop out. Now, we're talking about blisters and, of course, bleeding. I couldn't even do my exercises for my arm because of the blisters in my armpit.
>
> By this time, I began to really feel tired. Exhausted. And my ribs had started really hurting. The doctor said, "We had to go so deep with your radiation treatments that you have permanent damage now to your bone structure." That's why I'm sore through here (gestures to rib cage).

Although this woman had seen slides and read a booklet that mentioned burns and bone damage as possibilities, she felt she had not been adequately prepared for these side effects.

> I was not prepared for the burns. What they said on those slides was not adequate. It just blended in there. It's almost as if they want you to skip over it and not ask any questions about burns. Because if you did, you know what? You'd be as hesitant at taking radiology as I was chemotherapy. I felt angry, and I felt so disappointed!

(See also Ingrid's description of radiation in chapter 2.)

Chemotherapy

Chemotherapy is a systemic therapy used to destroy cancer cells throughout the body. It is usually used as an adjuvant, or secondary, therapy after the primary therapy (surgery) is complete. Until recently, chemotherapy has been used only for women who had positive lymph nodes removed during the surgery. The theory is that most patients with positive lymph nodes (Stage II cancers) will have distant micrometastases in other parts of the body. If not treated, these may become symptomatic sometime in the future. Once such metastases become symptomatic, they are usually no longer curable.

Some recent research also suggests that chemotherapy is effective in reducing the possibility of recurrence, even in women who have no positive lymph nodes (Stage I). Because most (70%) node-negative women do not experience recurrences, and because chemotherapy may prolong the lives of only about one third of those who do, routine chemotherapy for Stage I women is controversial. It means treating many women who will not benefit. Research is currently under way to determine which women will benefit, so the treatment can be targeted to them. There is also controversy surrounding the use of chemotherapy for older women, even those who have positive nodes. Some research has found that for these women, hormonal treatments are more effective.

Three major types of drugs are used to destroy cancer cells. These are called alkylating agents, antimetabolites, and antibiotics and are often used in combinations. These drugs serve to interfere with the process of cell division and growth. None can target only the cancer cells, however, so the process of cell division and growth is affected throughout the body, creating unpleasant side effects. These can include nausea, vomiting, and diarrhea; increased susceptibility to infection (because white blood cell production is reduced); hair loss; fatigue; weight gain; mouth ulcers; nervousness; and irritability. The number of these side effects and their severity varies from woman to woman, as does the ability to cope with them.

As with radiation, studies show that women undergoing chemotherapy have more psychological distress (Cooper, Cooper, & Faragher 1989; McArdle, Cooper, & Morran, 1979; Meyerowitz, Sparkes, & Spears, 1979; Penman et al., 1987; Tish-Knobf, 1986). This could be from the drugs themselves, or from the implication of being on chemotherapy (up until recently, needing chemotherapy meant that the cancer had spread beyond the breast).

In our study, most women were treated with adjuvant chemotherapy, but some refused it. One woman refused chemotherapy because she had had a course of chemotherapy after her lumpectomy, and it had not prevented a reccurrence. "I said it didn't work the first time, so why should I have it?" Another woman had watched a friend go through chemotherapy and later die. She adamantly refused chemotherapy herself, even though her cancer was advanced at the time of diagnosis. One node-negative woman, who rejected the option of chemotherapy, had a metastasis later and wondered if it could have been prevented with chemotherapy (see case study on Ingrid in chapter 2).

Chemotherapy has a very bad reputation, and most of the women in our sample experienced the common side effects. Although some were "wiped out" by the drugs, others were able to tolerate them fairly well. Some research has shown that most women have only mild symptom distress from chemotherapy (Tish-Knobf, 1986), and this seemed to be the case for many of the women we interviewed. Most found creative ways to cope, and many continued with very active lives throughout the treatment despite the side effects. Their ability to survive the chemotherapy seemed a source of pride for many women. The experiences of several women with chemotherapy are described subsequently.

> The first dosage didn't make me feel any differently at all. With the second dosage, my hair started falling out all over the place. Sores in my mouth. No nausea. It didn't stop me from doing anything I wanted to do, whether it was going down to the casino or going to a party. I took care of myself. I did take time in the afternoon to take a nap, and the majority of nights I'd say I was in bed by nine o'clock. But I continued teaching my aerobics classes. I wore a wig, because I lost it all [hair]. It came back in curly! I used to have to pay for this (gestures to her thick, curly hair)!
>
> Nancy, age 36

> I felt the chemotherapy was like being pregnant. I gained weight, I felt nauseous, I was hungry for strange things, I didn't look like myself, I couldn't wear my normal clothes.
>
> Lisa, age 37

> At one point during treatment, I lost my eyesight for about a half hour. That was scary. I had headaches. I would have this metallic taste in my mouth. My hair got thin, but I didn't lose it. I didn't go bald. I didn't have to wear a wig, because I have very thick hair. I never missed a day of work. I would have the drug around lunchtime, and then work until six. Then I would get home, and I'd help my daughter with her lessons and get her situated, and then, about eight o'clock at night, it would hit me, and I could do nothing. Raising my arm took everything I had. But the next morning, I was OK.
>
> Debra, age 39

(See case studies on Karen (chapter 2), Ruth and Laura (chapter 3), Sandra (chapter 4), and Judith (chapter 6) for further descriptions of chemotherapy.)

One reaction to chemotherapy that several women reported in our interviews was the cessation of menstruation and the symptoms of menopause. Although it is known that chemotherapy brings on menopause (sometimes only temporarily), in most premenopausal women (Tish-Knobf, 1986) this is not generally included in the lists of possible side effects given to women; many in our sample were not aware of it. In her account of her breast cancer experience, Eleanor Bergholz (1988) tells of her experience. "After the second [chemotherapy] treatment, my menstrual period stopped. . . . When I asked my oncologist, he said with a shrug, 'You may still get a period again or you may not. But be sure to use birth control because you certainly wouldn't want to get pregnant now that you've had cancer.' His expression seemed to say it was of no real concern, my abruptly having no more periods. Perhaps he had seen too much. After all, what is a period if it is cancer we are talking about?" (pp. 77–78)

Anne (age 39) says, "I've probably gone through menopause. I lost my period when I had chemotherapy. The older you are, the less chance of getting your period back if you lose it during chemotherapy. In my age group, it was like a 50:50 chance. Well, I never did. I went through hot flashes, and normal kind of wudgy (feeling bad)." Alice (age 43) says, "I had my last period when I started chemo, and I have never seen any signs of it since, not even a little pink spot. I dried up like a prune. I don't know if it was my chemistry or if the chemo made it happen" (see also case study on Sandra in chapter 4).

Many women also complained that chemotherapy put a damper on their sex lives (Meyerowitz et al., 1979; Silberfarb et al., 1980). Because of the various side effects, women undergoing chemotherapy often did not feel "in the mood" for sex. They were too tired, or they felt unattractive. We found a big difference in the resumption of sexual relations for those women whose surgery was followed by chemotherapy and those who did not have chemotherapy. With the new 1988 National Cancer Institute recommendations for even node-negative women to consider chemotherapy, we would anticipate increased problems in the sexual area. In our interviews, the chemotherapy seemed more of a hindrance to sexual activity than did the mastectomy. Sally (age 37) says, "That whole year, I didn't feel like having sex. Now, we really don't have much of a sex life. I think part of it is being out of the habit." As a result of her dissatisfaction with her lack of sexuality, another woman has decided to take estrogen replacements, even though she is afraid that this could contribute to a reccurrence of her cancer. "You put yourself at risk. It's hard. But there also has to be quality to life. It's not fair to keep somebody around and feel like a dried up old fish."

One interesting characteristic of chemotherapy is that it is often the only thing that makes a women actually feel ill. Most women feel no symptoms with their cancer. Even if they feel a lump, they do not experience "illness." They feel healthy. This feeling of health contrasts with the news that they have a very serious disease. When the chemotherapy begins, they actually begin to feel ill—not because of the disease but because of the treatment. Roberta expresses it this way. "I had a hard time believing that I was ill because I didn't feel that I was. I was never sick until I was taking medication to make me better. When I started [chemotherapy], that's when I started to feel bad and look horrible. That makes it even harder to go through."

Because the side effects of the chemotherapy are the first "sick" feelings a woman has, she may wonder if these symptoms are from the breast cancer rather than the chemotherapy. Renee, for example, whose cancer was discovered on a mammogram, had a mastectomy, followed by a course of chemotherapy. During the chemotherapy, she experienced some nausea, mouth sores, and tiredness. "Am I tired from the chemotherapy, or is it from the cancer continuing to grow inside?" she remembers thinking. Judith (age 64) (see case study in chapter 6) had some serious problems during the chemotherapy that she also interpreted as a possible spread of the cancer. It was not until the chemotherapy was over that these women were able to regain a feeling of health.

One positive side effect of intravenous chemotherapy is the social interaction that can result just from gathering a group of people with cancer together. Several women seemed almost to enjoy the chemotherapy sessions for this reason.

> When I would go in for [chemotherapy] treatments, it was set up like a beauty salon. You had the chairs and all the [intravenous] bags, and everybody sat in one group. It was just missing the hair dryers on the back of the chairs. You would see the same people, if you were on the same schedule. So it was, "Oh Hi! How are you doing?" You know, just as if you were going somewhere for anything else. It was very sincere. It was almost a social type of thing. It was not sterile at all.
>
> Roberta, age 32

> When that finished, it was sort of disconcerting not to be going to the oncology center every week, where they talked to you and you got to see people. People would just sort of sit and talk about the most incredible things. There was a bond!
>
> Lisa, age 37

> That year was a great year of camaraderie. I would go for the chemotherapy, and you'd sit there and see all these people, and they look so desperately ill. And you sit down with these people, and they had the best outlook on life. They were alive! They were the most kind, humane people. They were able to deal with it and talk about it. It was just great! They ended up being so positive for me.
>
> Deborah, age 39

In some settings, chemotherapy seems to provide a close support group. Perhaps like the groups formed under the stress of battle, people going through chemotherapy together also develop a close bond. Also, the knowledge that they are being closely monitored is comforting to many women, who may experience a sense of abandonment by the medical world when chemotherapy ends. Holland and Rowland (1987) conclude, "It is important to anticipate and plan for emotional reactions to ending treatment when, as with radiotherapy, fears of recurrence peak. Our clinical experience suggests that many women experience severe reactive anxiety and depression at this time, perhaps because of their greater awareness of relative survival statistics" (p. 642).

Hormone Therapy

It has been known for a long time that disrupting the cancer's supply of estrogen can cause the tumor to shrink. At one time, the ovaries of breast cancer patients were removed for this reason. Today, there is an antiestrogen drug, tamoxifen, which has few side effects. Another recent advance has been the development of laboratory tests that can determine, from the tissue taken in the biopsy, whether the tumor is estrogen or progesterone receptive—that is, whether it responds to these hormones by growing. If so, then an antiestrogen drug is likely to be effective in blocking tumor growth. Some research suggests that younger women do not benefit from hormone treatment, although this is controversial.

Marian (age 56) was put on estrogen for 5 years following her hysterectomy. Then, when breast cancer was discovered, she was taken off the estrogen and put on tamoxifen. She describes her reaction.

> I had a lot of attacks of just water—and I mean water! It just ran off me like someone was holding a spigot over me. I had heard of these things called hot flashes. I never felt hot, but it was horrifying because I could be sitting here with you and all of a sudden the water would just start running off me.

(See case studies on Laura in chapter 3 and Gwen in chapter 5) for further examples.)

Reconstruction

Breast reconstruction is more and more popular, as techniques improve and more insurance companies are covering the cost. In our study, 29% of the women interviewed had had reconstructive surgery, and several others were considering it, including several who had had mastectomies many years earlier. The commonest type of reconstruction uses a silicone implant, placed under the muscles of the chest or between the skin and the muscle. Sometimes the mastectomy scar can be used, so that the woman has only one scar. In some cases, an empty bag is inserted, and then is gradually inflated with injections of silicone or saline. Reconstruction can also be done using a "flap" of tissue from the woman's back or abdomen. Nipples and areolae can also be reconstructed, usually in a separate operation. Skin grafts are often used to accomplish this. Recently, tatooing is being used to simulate the darker skin of the areola.

The decision whether or not to have reconstruction varies from woman to woman. We found women at all ages deciding both ways. For example, one woman in her 60s had reconstruction, not because of cosmetics but because she had serious back problems, exacerbated by her mastectomy, which left her badly out of balance. An older single woman was considering reconstruction because she wanted to "feel like a woman." The decisions of younger women also varied. One woman in her 30s said, "I suppose I could get another *mound* if I wanted one," her coping mechanism of "minimizing" interfering with possible reconstruction. Most of the younger women did have reconstruction, however. (All of the women in our sample who had reconstruction had implants.)

Research on the effect of reconstruction is controversial (Boudreau, 1988; Freeman et al., 1984; Meyerowitz, Chaiken, & Clark, 1988), but most women have been found to be highly satisfied (Rowland et al., 1984). The women in our sample were also satisfied, although many expressed some disappointment at first (see case studies on Dorothy in chapter 2 and Jessica in chapter 4). Several women expressed disappointment that the implants have no feeling. All were pleased with how they looked in clothes, however, and were happy to be rid of the inconveniences of using a prosthesis. Maguire (1983) found that women "responded well to breast reconstruction providing they were realistic about the results that could be achieved, were aware of the possible complications, wanted a cleavage rather than a breast as good as the original, and wanted it for themselves and not because of pressure from others" (p. 81).

When to do the reconstruction is controversial. Some research shows that when reconstruction is done right after the mastectomy, women are spared the negative effect of mastectomy on body image and sexuality (Holland & Rowland, 1987; Schain, Wellisch, Pasnau, & Landsverk, 1985). Conversely, some plastic surgeons prefer to wait for 6 months to a year, until the body has healed from the mastectomy. Wendy (age 38) had a problem with a reconstruction that was done immediately. In the year following her operation, she experienced a substantial weight gain, as do many breast cancer patients.

> I put on over 20 pounds. That was really depressing, because I had been a really good size. I gained 4 lb a month for 6 months! What's really funny now is that because I've gained the weight, they're [breasts] not the same size [laughs]. When I went back to the plastic surgeon a year later, he was very unhappy with his work. "Oh, I don't think I put the right size [implant] in!" he said. I said, "No. It's not your fault. I put the weight on after the reconstruction, so the right one is bigger now."

PSYCHOSOCIAL ASPECTS OF BREAST CANCER

Parallel to the medical experiences described in the previous section, a woman with breast cancer will experience reactions at the psychological level and disruptions in her social relationships. It is well known that the diagnosis of any serious illness precipitates a crisis for the individual and for the family. A crisis is defined as a situation in which the steady state of the system is disrupted, and the usual coping or problem-solving mechanisms prove inadequate. Serious illness may mean loss of key roles, changes in appearance and, consequently, self-image, loss of control, and an uncertain future (Mailick, 1979). Psychological changes may include feelings of anxiety, anger, guilt, helplessness, and depression (Moos & Tsu, 1977). There may be a major disruption of existing goals, patterns of behavior, and beliefs (Schoenrich, 1971). "Catastrophic illness poses a major challenge not only to the person's physical well-being, but also to his or her sense of identity and the continuation or maintenance of existing social relationships" (Blazyk & Canavan, 1986, p. 20). In this section, we consider the psychological and social tasks with which women with breast cancer are confronted. The "breast cancer tasks" are identified as (a) managing psychological reactions, (b) preserving a satisfactory body image, (c) maintaining satisfactory sexual relationships, (d) adjusting to role shifts, and (e) dealing with an uncertain future.

Managing Psychological Reactions

There has been an extensive amount of research and discussion on the psychological reactions of breast cancer patients. The earliest research focused on the question: What is the rate of psychological disorder in breast cancer patients? Although some early studies showed that around one quarter to one third of women showed some psychiatric disorder after being treated for breast cancer (Maguire, 1983; Maguire et al., 1978), more recent studies suggest that whereas most women experience some depression, anxiety, and anger (Meyerowitz, 1980), the rate of actual pathology is no higher than for other women (Psychological Aspects of Breast Cancer Study Group, 1987; Vinokur, Threatt, Caplan, & Zimmerman, 1989; Worden & Weisman, 1977). Research has also looked into the timing of psychological reactions, with results showing the most difficult times to be while awaiting surgery (Romsaas, Malec, Javenkoski, Trump, & Wolberg, 1986), the period following surgery (Jamison, Wellisch, & Pasnau, 1978; Worden & Weisman, 1977), and at first recurrence (Silberfarb et al., 1980). Most studies show a gradual return to normal levels of anxiety and depression (Meyerowitz, 1980). One study, however, concluded that "difficulties in adjustment are not confined to the early phase" (Northouse, 1989, p. 511).

Virtually all of the women in our study experienced some anger, anxiety, and depression. As the research would predict, however, we saw very few cases in which the women had not resolved these feelings at the time of the interview. (Remember that we required women to be at least 1 year postdiagnosis to be included.) We also found that strong feelings tended to come up again for women in three situations. One was when being exposed to information about breast cancer. Many women indicated that reading about breast cancer, or hearing about other women who got breast cancer, had a recurrence, or died from breast cancer was very stressful. Anne (age 37), for example, says the following.

> I didn't want to read too much for fear I'd find out something I didn't want to know. One day, *Ladies Home Journal* comes and I see "Breast Cancer—What Every Woman Dreads." So you think I'm not going to read that? So I read it and I get all upset, and I think, "Why did I do this to myself?"

Going in for annual checkups and waiting for the results of tests taken at these appointments are also very stressful times.

> I go right from the office down to get the blood taken. I don't want to wait. They say I can't get the results for 4 days, even though the lab says they will be ready this afternoon! Then, on the 4th day, I sit by the phone. I know I'll go nuts if I don't make the call. I sit there with my hand on the phone. Then, after I call I usually have to wait for the doctor to call me back. It's awful! All this waiting!

Even Wanda, who has had 12 years since her diagnosis with no recurrence describes the constant fear.

> You always have that fear. You're terrified of recurrence. That's why you're afraid to go in for a checkup. The day I go in, I'm very anxious. I will worry as long as I live.

Another thing that raises anxiety for the woman who has had breast cancer is any physical symptom that she thinks might be a metastasis. Quint (1963) points out that "every ache and pain takes on a new, fearful meaning." As Laura (chapter 3) says, "You never have another innocent pain."

It is not uncommon for people faced with serious illness to experience self-absorption. It is normal for people to turn inward and to focus their energies on the disease. Many of the women in our study talked about wanting to be alone for a period. This was especially problematic for women who were mothers of young children (see discussion on adjusting to role shifts later in this chapter). Like the other psychological reactions, self-absorption occurs early in the disease and gradually declines.

Perhaps another way of wording "managing psychological reactions" is to say that cancer patients need to learn to strike some kind of a balance between hope and dread (Wiener, 1975). Even in the very advanced stages of cancer, it is still possible to hope—for a cure, for an easy death, for freedom from pain, or to reach specific milestones (such as the birthday of a child, a graduation, or a wedding). The opposite is also true. A patient whose cancer was discovered early, who had no lymph node involvement, and who has had no signs of recurrence can still be overwhelmed by dread over the possibility that the cancer might return. Although there is probably no such thing as too much hope, a woman who denies the serious aspects of her disease may not be compliant with medical recommendations. Conversely, every women needs to keep the level of dread in check to get on with her life.

What kind of coping mechanisms do women use to help them to find this balance? Most of the literature on coping with breast cancer emphasizes denial (Meyerowitz, Heinrich, Coscarelli & Schag, 1983; Polivy, 1977) ("I thought, 'This isn't really cancer. This is just something else' "). Other coping mechanisms we saw included minimizing the importance of the loss of the breast ("It seemed that the males around me were far more concerned with this mound of flesh than I was"); bargaining ("If the hospital would just send me a letter saying that they removed my breast by mistake, and I didn't really have cancer, I wouldn't even complain"); selective comparison ("It's not like losing an arm or a leg"); religion ("He said, 'Do you believe Christ died for you?' I said, 'Of course he did.' And this was the most miraculous thing that ever happened to me in my whole life. I wasn't afraid any more! I was instantly filled with peace"); humor ("One day at work, I put a pencil in my pocket, and it went through my breast [prosthesis], and it started to ooze, and I thought to myself, 'I bet none of you can do that!' "); refusal to accept future implications ("My husband would say, 'Well, we have to take each day at a time. We don't have to think too far in the future.' And so we go, day by day"); and rehearsal of alternative outcomes by purposely bringing themselves face to face with death ("I chose to make the journey [dying] with her").

Overall, we found a wide variety of coping styles, with most women using different ones at different times. Although recent literature suggests that denial is a particularly effective coping mechanism (Dean & Surtees, 1989; Meyerowitz et al., 1983), the women in our sample who relied heavily on denial seemed the most anxious. The heavy use of denial may also cut women off from some of the most effective forms of social support. For example, Anne (age 37), who uses denial heavily, will not attend a support group ("Groups are not for me. I don't need to rehash it. The more I can forget about it, the better off I am"). Roberta remembers how she reacted to people after her surgery. "I appreciated the people who would visit or talk or whatever but would not mention it at all. Because they knew I was feeling terrible, they didn't ask me how I felt. That way I didn't have to lie and say everything was wonderful. I didn't like it when people said, 'How are you feeling?' or 'This must be horrible for you.' That wasn't what I wanted or needed."

One coping mechanism used by almost all of the women in our sample was to focus on the benefits. So many women told how their experience with cancer had ultimately improved the quality of their lives. They had learned to refocus life onto the things that really mattered—their relationships with their families and friends—and to let go of the small problems that plague everyday life. These women had truly learned to "make lemonade" out of their experience with breast cancer.

Preserving a Satisfactory Body Image

Because of recent advances in surgical treatment, and the increasing use of breast reconstruction techniques, breast cancer does not assault the body image as much as it once did. Most of breast cancer patients still undergo mastectomy, however, and need to come to terms with this. Because the breast is highly valued as a part of feminine beauty in American society (Schain, 1977), its loss can be traumatic. The literature on body image in mastectomy patients is inconsistent. Some research shows that many mastectomy patients have body image problems (Carroll, 1981; Maguire, 1983), whereas other studies show this to be untrue (Krouse & Krouse, 1982). Meyerowitz et al. (1988) suggest that perhaps too much emphasis has been placed on appearance in breast cancer patients. It has also been suggested that whether or not a woman will experience problems with body image depends on whether her scar has to be revealed (Metzger, Rogers, & Bauman, 1983). It is true that many women in our sample experienced difficulty showing the mastectomy scar to partners. Conversely, most of the women emphasized that they were far more concerned about having cancer than they were about losing a breast (Alagaratnam & Kung, 1986). Fran, for example, says "The fact that I might die was more devastating to me than the thought of losing my breasts." Kate says it this way, "I never felt like the loss of the breast diminished me as a woman. If I had been run over by a car and hit my breast and it had to be removed, that would be fine. It was the idea that it was cancer that was the cause of the removal. In my mind, cancer was death."

Recent literature on characteristics of women choosing lumpectomy versus mastectomy indicates that those choosing lumpectomy place a higher value on physical appearance (Margolis et al., 1989; Wolberg et al., 1987). It seems likely too that women who highly value physical appearance would be more concerned about body image following mastectomy.

Debra (age 39) is an example of a woman who was divorced at the time of her mastectomy and worried about how she would look. She was very encouraged by meeting the Reach to Recovery volunteer. "It was the best thing in the world. The girl was younger than me. She had bilateral mastectomies, and she looked *good!*" Later, Debra tells how she learned that she was still attractive to men after her mastectomy.

> One of the things that really made me feel good was there was a big dance, and I had a girlfriend make me a dress. I designed this dress, and it came across the shoulder, and it was kind of slinky. It was black. I borrowed a girlfriend's mink coat. It was *stunning!* I got so much attention from the men that were there. And I realized that *no one knew!*

Maintaining Satisfactory Sexual Relationships

Closely related to "preserving a satisfactory body image" is "maintaining satisfactory sexual relationships." The literature suggests that about one quarter to one third of mastectomy patients develop sexual problems (Maguire 1978, 1983), and that the sexual adaptation was related to the quality of the relationship before the illness (Woods & Earp, 1978). Schain (1988) points out that sexuality is an area that tends to be neglected by physicians. The women in our study reflected this point. Those who experienced chemotherapy were generally not warned that the treatment might result in menopause and a decreased libido. One woman, whose plastic surgeon used part of the nipple on her remaining breast to construct a nipple for her reconstructed breast, was not told that the loss of all sensation in the remaining part of the nipple was a possible side effect. She was quite disappointed to find that she now had no feeling in either nipple (see case study on Ruth in chapter 3). As mentioned earlier, many women expressed disappointment that the reconstructed breast had no feeling. Nor are physicians alone guilty in neglecting this area. Women in support groups, cancer support organizations like Reach to Recovery, and even psychotherapy told us repeatedly that sexuality had never been discussed!

In our sample, most women returned to their previous level of sexual activity fairly soon. Those who had chemotherapy or hormonal treatment, however, often suffered severe disruption of their sex lives. Women were not always able to reactivate sexuality after treatment ended. The reaction of husbands or partners seemed to be very important. The two lesbian women in our sample indicated that they thought breasts were less important to them than to heterosexuals. They did not report problems resuming sexual activities.

Sexual intimacy for a single women who is not in a serious relationship means having to tell potential partners and to face their reactions. Debra shares the following experience.

> We started dating in August, and eventually, he started hinting about going away for a weekend together. And I thought, "God! The man has not seen this. I don't know if I can handle this. What am I going to do?" So one night, when he was saying good night, I said, "Remind me to tell you something some day." He turned to me and said, "Tell me now." So I told him. Well, I thought he was going to cry. He just welled up, and he couldn't speak for a while. Then he said, "Oh, I'm just so sorry to hear that. Do you want me to see it now?" I said, "No, I'm not prepared to do this now." He said, "Fine." And, in time, we ended up having a physical relationship. It ended up that it was not a problem for him, so it was not a problem for me.

Debra's example, like many women in our sample, shows that although women may be very fearful of rejection, this is a hurdle that can be surmounted. In case after case, men were able to show their wives or lovers that they still loved and cherished them (see case studies on Beth and Jessica in chapter 5). One wonderful husband told his wife (who was going through chemotherapy) that he found her baldness very sexy!

Adjusting to Role Shifts

Sickness, almost by definition, means an inability to perform social roles (Parsons & Fox, 1952). Penman et al. (1987) found that breast cancer patients had more difficulty than controls carrying out social roles, but that the differences disappeared within 1 year. With breast cancer, the physical disability depends on the treatments. For those with surgical removal of lymph nodes in the armpit area, there is a postsurgical period when normal activities may be disrupted. Many of the women complained about not being able to drive. Several were unable to play sports, like tennis, which involve lifting of the arm. For women who undergo a course of chemotherapy or radiation, the side effect of tiredness can seriously limit normal activities. Even for women who do not experience these treatments, however, the psychological effects can be disruptive. Depression, for example, involves a loss of interest in normal activities (see case study on Judith in chapter 6).

Because women are usually nurturers of their families, self-absorption can mean a turning away from important social roles. One mother said, "I totally forgot about my daughter. I was so wrapped up in myself." Several women who were mothers of young children sent the children to stay with grandparents, feeling that they just couldn't "be there" for them at this point. For example, Lily sent her 18-month-old daughter to stay with her parents. "I *had* to do it; I couldn't care for myself and her too. I had to learn about it [breast cancer]. I couldn't concentrate on anything else. Nothing. Even when I did visit her, I wasn't sure I was there. I could only concentrate on myself."

Mothers of adolescent children may turn to these children for support, and this can disrupt normal relationships (see chapter 5 for discussion of adolescent children). In marriages where the woman has been the main provider of emotional support, a shift in marital roles may occur (see chapter 5 for discussion of marriage).

Because most women today are working, there is also the possibility for disruption of the work role. In our sample, however, there were few major work disruptions. Most women missed some work but were proud of how successfully they were able to continue. Nancy, for example, continued to teach her aerobic dance class through her chemotherapy. ("It didn't stop me from doing anything I wanted to do.") Even the women who did not work outside the home were eager to return to their responsibilities. Edith, for example (chapter 6), tells how her husband helped with the housework after her surgery but didn't "baby her," and she took on these responsibilities as soon as she could.

In our sample, the work disruptions were more due to women refocusing their lives (see chapters 2, 3, and 5) than to physical problems. Work may also be affected in that women who have had breast cancer may experience employment discrimination (McCharen & Earp, 1981) and may be reluctant to change jobs in the future because of difficulties getting health insurance. (This did not come up in our sample, perhaps because most of our interviews took place fairly soon after diagnosis.)

Dealing with an Uncertain Future

There was a time when surgeons would reassure breast cancer patients that they were sure they had removed all of the cancer. This reassurance was based on the theory that cancer began in the breast, then spread to nearby areas, and finally spread to distant parts of the body. According to this theory, survival rates should be improving, because with increased use of breast self-examination and mammogram, breast lumps are being detected earlier and earlier, and these cancers are being removed when they are small. Survival rates have not declined significantly, however, despite earlier detection. New theories of breast cancer suggest that some women may have a type of tumor that spreads very rapidly—even before the tumor can be detected in the breast. Other women may have very slow-growing tumors that may never spread beyond the breast (Boston Women's Health Collective, 1976; Fisher & Barboni, 1982). According to this more systemic theory of breast cancer, no woman can be reassured that all the cancer was removed with surgery. Even in Stage I breast cancer, it is possible that very small cancer cells have spread to other parts of the body. The result of these newer theories is that no woman with breast cancer can be certain that she will not experience a recurrence or a metastasis. Anne (age 37) tells how she experiences this uncertainty. "My doctor is very straight with me. He says, 'Your chances are very good.' But they don't know. They'll never say, 'You're cancer free.' That would sound so good to a person. But they don't do that. They can't." Lisa (age 37) talks about no longer having a long-term perspective.

> It occurred to me that I no longer had a long-term perspective. I remember after law school when I'd go for interviews, people would say, "What do you expect to be doing in 5 or 10 years?" Now, I get angry when people start talking as if they can plan their lives that way. I got roped into planning a 10th reunion for my college. And the chairman said, "When you have the reunion, you should choose a reunion chairman for 5 years from now." And I thought, "What an imposition!" You know, to expect that somebody would have to be around in 5 years to be the reunion chairman! Maybe [the woman from the class of] 1929 was thinking about that, too.

Lisa, who had one small child, also decided not to have any more children after her diagnosis.

> If I hadn't gotten breast cancer, I probably would have seriously thought about having another child. I don't know if we would have, but it was an option. As soon as I was diagnosed, I said—"Uh-oh. No more kids." Because I really thought that it would be a terrible imposition to have a child when you don't know what was going to happen to you.

Wendy, also age 37, tries not to think of the possibility of death. "You can look at it and say, 'I'm not going to buy another house, 'cause that's a whole new mortgage and I don't know if I'm going to be here in 5 years.' But you can't do that. You can't let it ruin your life."

Debra uses her religion to help her deal with an uncertain future. "I had to learn that the Lord isn't going to give me any less or any more days than I'm supposed to have. Worrying about it isn't going to make it any better. He already knows when He's going to take me home."

Most of the women in our sample used the knowledge of their uncertain futures to refocus their lives onto the things that were important to them, and to let go of the less important things, like daily hassles or material things. For most, this meant focusing on the important people in their lives—husbands, children, lovers, and friends. It also meant devoting more time to themselves and really enjoying their lives (see case studies for numerous examples). Knowing that their time might be limited made most of them value—just living—and making the most of the time they did have.

Social Support

In her ground-breaking book, Gilligan (1982b) points out that women's conceptions of self are rooted in a sense of connection and relatedness to others. Women with breast cancer make use of their relationships with others to help them master the illness tasks of managing psychological reactions, preserving a satisfactory body image, maintaining satisfactory sexual relationships, adjusting to role shifts, and dealing with an uncertain future. There is an increasing amount of literature that shows that psychosocial and medical outcome of breast cancer is related to social support (Bloom, 1982; Bloom & Spiegel, 1984; Friedman et al., 1988; Levy, Herberman & Winkelstein, 1987; Levy et al., 1990; Neuling & Winefield, 1988; Penman et al., 1987; Spiegel, Bloom, Kraemer, & Gottheil, 1989; Zemore & Shepel, 1989).

    Although there is some literature suggesting that friends and acquaintances withdraw from the seriously ill (Wortman & Dunkel-Schetter, 1979) studies on women with breast cancer suggest that for most women, levels of social support are high (Smith, Redman, Burns, & Sagert, 1985; Zemore & Shepel, 1989). The husband is the most important source of support for married women, followed by other family and friends (Holland & Rowland, 1987).

    Many women in our sample talked with tremendous feeling about the importance to them of all forms of the social support they received, including small things like receiving cards and flowers. In our culture, women tend to be providers of social support rather than receivers. The experience of receiving support was a delightful change for many of them. One woman reports that one of her fondest memories is the birthday party her family gave her after her diagnosis.

> My 45th birthday was the nicest I ever had. I came home around nine, and they had a birthday cake with candles on it and cards. They were very sweet for about a half-an-hour [laughs]. It was very special. For 30 minutes, they paid attention to me!

This example shows not only the increased support but how rare it has been for this woman to receive it.

    Not all women were comfortable with the increased support. Dorothy, for example (chapter 3), didn't want to feel helpless. Many of the women in our study stayed in a caregiver role, even as they went through the worst moments of the breast cancer experience. Women of all ages tended to think of the needs of others first, and tried to protect and support their loved ones at a time when they themselves needed protection and support. Examples include Karen (age 28) (chapter 2), who made sure her mother was not alone when she received the news of Karen's cancer; Audrey (age 40), a nun who called her coworkers from the recovery room after her mastectomy to reassure them that she was all right; and Theresa (age 70), who tells the following story.

> I have been healthy most of my life. And when he [husband] would have to change my dressings, he was crying. You are talking about a chest here that's all scarred, and now its burnt and blistered too. He'd reach over and kiss me and he'd say, "Hang in there, kid. We're going to see this through." And then I would cry because he was crying and I thought, "My God, it isn't fair to put him through all of this!"

Because of the importance of social connectedness to women, we will examine the impact of breast cancer on key social relationships through the life course. Relationships with husbands, lovers, children, parents, and friends are explored in the context of life-course development.

Life Stage and Breast Cancer

It is the thesis of this book that women in different stages of life-course development experience breast cancer in different ways. In this chapter, we have focused on some of the universals in the experience. The following chapters, in contrast, each deal with a separate life stage. In each chapter, several case studies are presented that are representative of women in the particular life stage, and then several themes are explored that we thought were central to that life stage.

In the breast cancer literature, age has been considered primarily as a possible predictor of psychosocial outcome. That is, the question that has been asked is: Which are better off—older or younger women? The research results have been equivocal. Some studies indicate that breast cancer is more traumatic for younger women (Hughson, Cooper, McArdle, & Smith, 1988; Jamison et al., 1978; Penman et al., 1987; Smith et al., 1985; Vinokur et al., 1989), whereas others report mixed results (Holland & Mastrovito, 1980; Holland & Rowland, 1987; Metzger et al., 1983); no differences (Bloom, 1982); and that older women had more problems with it (Goin & Goin, 1981; Kushner, 1975). This research is problematic for several reasons. First, it has no clear theoretical framework. Theory tends to be applied only later, to explain the findings. When the results show that younger women have more problems, the speculation is that younger women are more invested in their bodies and have less experience dealing with crisis. When older women seem to have more problems, the speculation is that they define cancer as a threat to life, or they have suffered more losses and are more prone to depression. Another problem is that age is considered as a continuous variable, and most statistical methods used are based on the assumption of linear relationships. This hardly makes conceptual sense, and it makes it very difficult to see if the most problematic age is somewhere in the middle of the continuum.

We would like to raise a different question, focusing not on which group is better off, but on how life stage and breast cancer interact, and on how this interaction affects the experience of breast cancer for women in each age group. We suspect not that women in one stage adjust better than another, but that women in different stages experience breast cancer differently, focus on different issues, and attach different levels of importance to different aspects of the experience. The remainder of this book explores this thesis.

meaning is influenced by life stage.

2 Experiencing Breast Cancer in Young Adulthood: The Twenties

The case studies of three women (Rosemary, Karen, and Ingrid) are examples of how breast cancer impacts on the lives of women in their 20s. Their stories provide a rich account of how both single and married young women cope with breast cancer. Rosemary, a single 26-year-old woman had a steady boyfriend and worked at a hospital coordinating volunteer programs at the time of her diagnosis. Following a modified, radical mastectomy, Rosemary discovered she was pregnant and underwent an abortion before beginning chemotherapy. One year later Rosemary elected breast reconstruction. Karen was 28, single, and working as a speech therapist during the day while she attended school at night when she was diagnosed with breast cancer. After securing a second opinion, Karen elected a modified, radical mastectomy followed by chemotherapy and breast reconstruction. Ingrid, a 28-year-old woman, had been married for 8 years and was working as a health educator when her breast cancer was diagnosed. Ingrid had a lumpectomy (negative lymph nodes) followed by 10 weeks of radiation treatment. One year later, a biopsy of Ingrid's lung revealed a metastasis for which surgery was not indicated. Ingrid discovered she was pregnant during this time and had to have an abortion before beginning chemotherapy.

These three case studies illustrate the themes that emerged from our interviews as being most important for women with breast cancer in this phase of life. Rosemary, Karen, and Ingrid had all physically moved away from their parents' home at the time of diagnosis and were struggling to "achieve independence" while adjusting to new dependency needs brought on by coping with breast cancer. The issue of "fertility" was prominent in the stories of all three women as they concerned themselves with issues of bearing children and having breast cancer. One major goal of the 20s is "developing intimate relationships." All three young women struggled to form new relationships and preserve ongoing intimate relationships as they dealt with the issues of breast cancer. Most young adults are working on "finding a place in the adult world" as they attempt to actualize their dreams and ambitions. Both Rosemary and Karen focused on the career path in their 20s, whereas Ingrid focused on both marriage and work. In this chapter, these four themes (achieving independence, fertility, developing intimate relationships, and finding a place in the adult world) are examined as they relate to the breast cancer tasks.

CASE 1: ROSEMARY

Rosemary is a single woman, 26 years old. She has a mother, father, three younger siblings, and a steady boyfriend. One day, at a routine doctor's appointment, she mentioned that she had some pain in her chest, and could feel a small lump. She did not think of cancer but thought she may have strained a muscle while rearranging her furniture. The doctor (a general practitioner) thought it might be a clogged milk duct and tried a round of antibiotics. When that was unsuccessful, the doctor recommended a biopsy.

> Having a biopsy meant needles, and I was the worst person with needles, a real baby. I would cry at the thought. The biopsy was performed and when she [the surgeon] came back, I was told I had carcinoma of the breast. The first thing I thought about was my mortality. "Am I going to die?" She says "No, no, but you need surgery as soon as possible. The cancer is spreading at a very rapid rate." I could not choose a lumpectomy. It was out of the question. A modified radical mastectomy was my only option, with chemotherapy to follow. I wanted a second opinion, so I took all mammogram and chest x-rays to another hospital specialist. The diagnosis did not change. It was cancer.

Rosemary's mother and sister accompanied her to the hospital 2 weeks later for the surgery. During her hospital stay, Rosemary had lots of support from her family.

> Everybody was real supportive. I have a host of cousins and aunts and nieces and nephews too. When this happened, we decided not to tell them, so they wouldn't worry. We were going to tell them when I got out of the hospital, but somehow they found out. One of my aunts walked all the way to the hospital in really chilly weather. And she says, "You didn't tell us that you were in here, but we found out, and I'm here." And you know, from that day on she was there every day. She is just the sweetest person. You couldn't stop her from coming to the hospital to see me. All my family was really, really strong. My mom never showed her fear, but that's how moms are. I'm quite sure she cried a lot and prayed a lot too, but she didn't cry with me. I cried. I cried on her shoulder a lot, but she was being strong for me.

Following the surgery, Rosemary decided to stay by herself in her apartment—a decision that she regrets making.

> A lot of the sadness didn't hit me until I was home, because I live by myself. Mom said, "Oh, you can come stay here, you can stay at the house." I didn't want to—I wanted to be home. But maybe it would have been better if I was, you know, with my mom and my brothers and sister, even though they came to visit me. Every day I had the company of friends, but at night you have time to really think about things. I remember looking out the window at 4:30 in the morning, and there was nothing going by, just quiet, and thinking about myself. I was just so worried about me. I was 26 years old!

Rosemary had two major worries. One was that she had been told she should have chemotherapy. Not only did she harbor a real fear of needles, but chemotherapy brought back painful memories.

> What I remember about chemotherapy from being younger was my grandmother, who had cancer. She was on chemotherapy, and I just remember her pain, and her hair loss. Finally she passed away. And I said, "Chemotherapy didn't help her, is it going to help me?"

Rosemary's other concern was that she skipped her period following the mastectomy. She had her doctor check and found out that she was pregnant.

> I . . . they had to abort the baby. They wouldn't let me carry a child. There was a dilemma. If I had chemotherapy, there was a good chance the baby was going to die, or be deformed. And if I didn't have chemotherapy, they still felt there was a chance that I would die. That was a big loss, as well as a big shock for me.

During the period following her surgery, Rosemary remembers facing the loss of her breast.

> My mom changed the bandages for me for the first week, because I couldn't— I just couldn't bear to look at myself. Finally, one day in the shower, I thought, "I'm going to change the bandages myself." So finally I got up enough nerve to change them. It took me a week. I sat on the edge of the tub and cried again. I mourned for the loss of my breast. It's part of your femininity, so you mourn the loss.

Rosemary did finally agree to the chemotherapy, after her initial resistance.

> I finally broke down and said, "Okay, I'll go through with it." And I never asked anybody to go with me—I don't know why. Maybe it was my way of saying "I'm going to beat this thing."

Rosemary was feeling very "down" during her 6 months of chemotherapy. She had nausea and some hair loss, although "not as traumatic as my grandmother's had been."

That was just such a really depressing time. I could not sleep. I would be up all night, just walking and pacing and looking out the window. Finally, I asked for sleeping pills. I never thought I was going to make it through.

During this period, Rosemary stopped all physical exercise including her postmastectomy exercises.

I just stopped trying. I'd say "Oh, I don't have to do all these exercises." I really didn't try as much as I should have. The muscles of my arm started to shrink from nonuse. I was babying it. I was being a big baby, I guess, at the time. One of the things I would say was, "I'm going to die anyway, so what difference does it make?" So finally, they sent me to physical therapy. I had a wonderful doctor, so optimistic and full of life. I just needed a push. I started doing my exercises again, and I got my full range-of-motion back really really fast.

One of the things that helped Rosemary conquer her depression was her involvement in a support group.

It's needed. It really is. You need to talk to people. You can talk to your family—me and my mom had talked often—but if you haven't been there, you can feel sorry, you can sympathize, but you don't really understand. You haven't experienced it. So you need to talk to people who have experienced it.

Rosemary's boyfriend was supportive through this period.

I was very moody, very selfish. "I'm sick. I'm going to be sick, and if you don't like me being sick, that's your problem!" He stuck with me the whole time and dealt with my moodiness. Later, he told me, "You were very bitchy to me at that time in your life. I'm glad that's over with."

During chemotherapy, Rosemary's sex drive was "nil." Later she described some changes in her sex life.

I was on the pill, and then, after the diagnosis, the first thing they said was no more birth control pills. So then there's a dilemma—what are you going to do? My boyfriend and I used to have intercourse whenever we were in the mood. Now I have to get fitted for a diaphragm. . . . With diaphragms you can't be that spontaneous in your lovemaking. So that caused a problem. . . . The first couple of times I'm in the bathroom with the gel, and the diaphragm is bouncing—it was so funny [laughing]—the diaphragm is bouncing all over the place until I got the hang of it, and that was kind of frustrating. . . . So that put a little damper on things.

Another problem for Rosemary was her body image.

You just don't feel that sexy. Whoever thought of a sexy one-breasted person? I didn't feel comfortable being completely nude, so I wore a lot of different things to cover it up—T-shirts, camisoles, his shirts. He didn't mind. He understood. But that psychological block kept me from being completely uninhibited.

Rosemary bought an expensive prosthesis, but never felt comfortable with it and never wore it. About a year after her mastectomy, Rosemary decided to have reconstruction.

> At first, I was able to put myself in that category of "I don't care what society thinks, if I have to go around with one breast, I'll go around with one breast. If you don't like it, that's your problem." But then, after a year or so, I said, "My bathing suit doesn't fit right; my clothes don't really look right; maybe I'll get reconstruction."

Rosemary had four separate surgeries before the reconstruction was complete. She had an implant put in, which was then gradually filled with a saline solution to stretch the skin.

> I had an overinflated chest. I looked like a 36D on one side and 32B on the other! But now, I'm pretty happy that I had it done. It makes a whole difference in my outlook. It gives me a better self-image.

Looking back, Rosemary feels that her experience with cancer changed her in several positive ways.

> I'm more outgoing now than I was 3 or 4 years ago. I wasn't a totally reclusive type of person, but I was a pretty quiet person, and now I think I'm more assertive. I speak my mind—I've learned to say no, when I really just *don't want to do* something. People pull at you from all ends and you try to make different commitments, and you finally say, "I need a day for me. No, I can't do this." Instead of feeling *obligated* to do everything for everybody all the time, I have learned to pick and chose what I *want* to do. Yeah, it's been positive for me. It also gave me more confidence in the job that I had at that time. I became more outgoing, and work was so much more pleasurable.
>
> I just felt like this is not going to be the end of the world, that there's life after cancer. I guess inwardly I said, "I'm going to show people that I'm not a sickly person. You won't have to whisper the big C. Because with all the medical technology there is now, people are surviving."

Rosemary also attributes her recent job change to her experience with cancer.

> My diagnosis with breast cancer changed me, because I always thought I would be in the insurance world forever. I liked it—it paid well—but after I got involved with the support group I got this urge to help other people. . . . If I had to do it all over again, I'd be a doctor. If I could go back to high school and decide my path, it would be medicine. It really would.

Now 30 years old, Rosemary is working full-time in a hospital, coordinating volunteer programs. She and her boyfriend have separated.

> I still hope to marry some day. My life has not hit its peak yet, but I feel it will. However I will always have a fear and that is, "Will I be a good mother?" If I raise my children the way my mother and father raised me it'll be fine. But

there is a monkey wrench in there, because I am the first one in my family diagnosed with breast cancer. And that is something to think about when you are going to have children because they may at some time in their lives have breast cancer. Do I want to bring a child into this world and have them suffer the way I did? There was a lot of pain, anger, sorrow, frustration, and uncertainty at that point in my life. I still have time; my biological clock hasn't ticked out yet.

Overall, Rosemary maintains a positive outlook. In talking about living with the fear of recurrence, she says the following.

You wrestle with it. In my case, I come in contact with people who have had recurrences. You hope you don't have to go through it. And they say if you get through 5 years without a reoccurrence, you have a good chance of not having cancer ever again. I don't dwell on it, but I know in the back of my head there's always that possibility. You just hope that the Lord is going to get you through. My basic thing is we are healthy functioning people. Life goes on. You expand and you grow. Life is full of obstacles, and this is one of them. It's no reason to think that life is over for you. And for me, life is still just beginning.

CASE 2: KAREN

Karen, like so many young women today, has focused on building her career as a major focus of her 20s. At age 28, she was working full-time as a speech therapist in a New York hospital during the day and working on her master's degree at night. She lived alone in a small apartment and enjoyed spending her leisure time with several good friends. She is the middle of seven sisters, most of whom lived within a 3-hour drive. Karen's parents were divorced, and her father lived out of state. She had recently broken up with a man whom she had dated for quite a while. "I had not started dating anybody else, because I really wasn't ready to do that."

One day, she was taking a shower and found a lump in her breast. Because she was so young and had just had a complete gynecological examination (including a breast examination) 6 months earlier, her initial reaction was to try to deny that it was a lump. She also thought cancer was unlikely because there was no history of any kind of cancer in her family. She asked her sister, however, to "feel it just to see if she felt anything." She also felt a lump. So Karen knew that she had to do something about it. Her gynecologist tried to aspirate it twice, but nothing came out. "I knew it was not a good sign, but she [the gynecologist] kept trying to reassure me that I was too young to have any major problem." From that point on things happened very quickly—first a mammogram, then a surgical biopsy. The surgeon had told her to call for the results in a week, but, as she was getting off the table from the biopsy he said, "No you'd better come in on Monday." This made her think the tumor was probably cancer, and she spent the weekend preparing herself for bad news.

As she suspected, the biopsy result showed cancer, and her surgeon recommended a mastectomy.

> I went in and he told me it was a cancerous tumor. He was absolutely wonderful to me. He brought out pictures and showed me about the incision and about reconstruction right away. And he presented it in a positive way, if you can say anything is positive in having to have a mastectomy. We talked about it a little bit. He could see that I was upset. I was crying.

Karen called a friend to pick her up but waited until she had "worked it through a little bit" before calling her family.

> I called one of my sisters, the one I'm closest with, to tell her first. My mom lived by herself, and I didn't want to tell her when she was by herself.

When her mother learned about her daughter's cancer she was quite upset, but "having raised seven daughters, she's not the kind of person that falls apart." Later when Karen and her mother were talking, her mother said, "I would much rather it were me than you."

Following the biopsy, Karen saw another surgeon for a second opinion. He also recommended mastectomy.

> They did say that I could have a lumpectomy or a mastectomy, but at that time the long-term studies hadn't been published yet for people my age. And to be perfectly honest, if it happened again today, I would still go for the mastectomy, because I don't 100% believe all the studies of equality between lumpectomy and mastectomy. I just feel like a new cancer could show up in the same breast, and I would end up having a mastectomy later. I didn't like having breast cancer, and I didn't like the idea of having a mastectomy, but I didn't feel there was any choice.

Karen decided to have the mastectomy and was scheduled to enter the hospital just 2 weeks after her first visit with the gynecologist. During the week following her biopsy, Karen also had to deal with a very concerned family—"everybody wanted to come to the city."

> But I decided that wasn't going to be the best thing for me, nor for them. My mom was working at the time. All my sisters back home had families, and my sister in college would want to come and, you know . . . and so I just needed some time to get my act together and decide—process all this stuff.

Karen used the week before surgery to "take care of herself."

> I didn't know how people were going to react to me, and I wasn't prepared for reactions that might be negative. So I just felt that I needed to have time for myself. I live here by myself, but I have wonderful friends, and you just find

out how people will drop anything and just be with you. I spent a number of the days by myself and some of them getting together with people, or having people come over in the evening. You know, just talking, and making sure what I needed and what I didn't need. It was a good time for me to process stuff, but it was also nice to see who your true friends are . . . and that they're not turned off by cancer.

Karen did allow her family to come to her apartment 2 days before she was scheduled for surgery. Three sisters came with their husbands and children. Her mother came as well.

They ended up sleeping on the floor, and my mom went to stay with another friend that lived in the area. . . . My college roommate came down. . . . It was Saturday night that they came and we had this big dinner—about 14 people.

Karen's mother stayed in New York during the week that Karen was in the hospital for her mastectomy, but Karen was uncomfortable with her mother's wish to be around her so much.

I just felt like—"You don't have to just sit here and look at me the whole day! Like go to Fifth Avenue and go shopping." So I told her [in] little ways to get out. . . . I think there would be nothing worse than to have to sit in the hospital looking at me all day. She'd want to come in, but I didn't want her to have to sit there all the time. That was not necessary.

In addition to trying to reassure her family that she was OK, Karen also found herself being supportive and showing her friends how to handle the situation.

A lot of people don't know how to react. Like a friend of mine who came to visit me in the hospital started talking about the movie *Tootsie*. She was telling some funny part about breasts or something like that, and she told me later that she went out of the room and said to her husband, "I can't believe I said that!" I said, "What do you mean? I don't want you to treat me differently because I've had breast cancer. You can yell at me the same—tell me the same dirty jokes, or whatever. I want to be treated the same!"

When she first woke up following the surgery, she remembers feeling "wiped out" from the anesthesia, and immobilized from the bandages but in no pain. Her attitude was, "I'm not staying in these pajamas! I want to be up and dressed and walking around in normal clothes!" She began rehabilitation exercises as soon as she could. Also, she wanted to see her incision. "I'm kind of curious. I just wanted to see what it looked like."

The hardest part for me was that I couldn't bathe myself 100%, and I couldn't wash my hair. My friends would rotate doing it for me. And it worked, but it was a bit messy! Plus I'm right handed, and it was on my right side, so eating was hard to do.

Karen remembers a volunteer from Reach to Recovery coming to see her in the hospital.

> They must have thought I was 68 instead of 28, and they sent an older woman. The information she gave me was good, but she couldn't really talk to me much about being young and single, and having cancer in this day and age.

During the course of the chemotherapy, Karen felt tired but was able to return to work.

> I worked full-time, and I'd get chemo on my lunch hour, and then go back to work. Some days when I felt really crappy after chemo, I would stay home from work. But I found those days almost harder to deal with than going to work and feeling lousy, because at least work kept my mind off feeling sick.

Like many women, Karen lost about half of her hair during the chemo treatments.

> I have very thick hair, and if you didn't know me, you wouldn't be able to tell. Still, it was very traumatic for me—that experience of pulling hair out, brushing your hair and having a handful of hair come out in your hand. It made me feel very afraid. It was hard for me because people weren't very empathetic. I ended up cutting my hair 'cause I had really long hair, and I was afraid the weight was going to help pull it out.

Karen did not date during the time that she was going through chemo because "first of all I was feeling tired, and it would be hard to explain all that to some new man. I really didn't feel like dating, but I did do things to make myself physically look attractive. I had a different hairstyle, and I made sure I always wore makeup." Karen reported with a lot of feeling that what she would have liked during this time was the following.

> You really need to be in a relationship to get this, to have somebody to hold me, to cuddle, and that kind of stuff. You know, the physical affection, not really intercourse. That wasn't important to me *at all;* it was really just the physical affection that really, I think, can make a big difference.

Although Karen decided before her mastectomy to have reconstruction as soon as possible, she had to wait a year for the operation. So, one of the first things she did after leaving the hospital was to arrange to get a prosthesis.

> In the meantime [before the fitted prosthesis was ready] I wore a bra with the temporary prosthesis the Reach to Recovery visitor gives you in the hospital. I wore a shirt that was a little bit loose, but not too loose. I knew [laughing] people were going to be looking, trying to decide which side it was. I sort of made it a game to watch people try to be nonchalant—to try to look but not make it obvious that they're looking. I got a great kick out of that! I was

initially under the impression that I was going to need all these different kinds of clothes, or bras, but you really don't. The prosthesis fit in my bra really well, and didn't ride up or anything. So the heck with that stuff.

Karen had a prosthesis made that was the type that could be attached to her skin, a feature that she made use of when wearing a bathing suit.

I went to get fitted. I didn't realize how different breasts were. It took a while to get one that matched and that fit really well. I got the kind with a nipple-areolar complex. I could wear tight shirts, and I looked the same. I didn't feel self-conscious at all! The only thing that was difficult with my prosthesis was trying to get bathing suits. The worst thing is they have [laughing] what I call "old women" bathing suits for people with mastectomies. They are the big flowered type with skirts. It's just not a young person's type of bathing suit. It missed the boat. So I finally found a regular kind of bathing suit that would be okay with my prosthesis.

During Karen's chemotherapy treatment, her father died very suddenly of a heart attack—his death was more upsetting to Karen than she expected.

During that year there were three deaths—that year was horrible. A friend of mine, who was sort of like an adopted father, died in February; my grandfather died in April; and then my father died in August.

So many losses coupled together make for a much more complex grief reaction. Karen was only beginning to mourn the loss of her breast when she endured the death of her "adopted father," then her grandfather, and then her father. At this point, Karen entered therapy for a couple of months, because she felt like all her emotions were "on overload." "It was just too much—too many emotional things to deal with." She describes herself as having a difficult time dealing with not being able to do the things that she felt she should be able to do. "I couldn't keep up with all the volunteer work I did and go out with my friends, go to school—that kind of stuff. I needed permission to say 'no.' And it was helpful for a while. I got what I needed."

Although Karen found most people reacted very well, she also had to learn to say "no" to some people who she felt were "badgering" her with questions.

It probably takes about 2 years to really feel like you've got it all together again. Before that, sometimes you just don't feel like talking. And people may think they are helping you, but they can really hurt you badly. Sometimes I wanted to tell people to "bug off! You don't need to know everything." I had to learn to know when to say "No, I don't want to talk about it now."

One year following her mastectomy, Karen had an implant type of breast reconstruction, and 6 months later, she had the nipple reconstructed, using a graft from the groin. For Karen, there was no discomfort following the implant surgery, "because you can't really feel." She did have pain from the graft, however. "That was the worst part. I walked around like I'd just gotten off a horse for 2 weeks!" Karen was initially disappointed with the reconstruction because it didn't meet her expectations.

It wasn't until after her reconstruction that Karen began dating again. At first she was afraid to think about dating again—"What are men going to—how are men going to react to my having cancer?" Karen's first dating experience after her mastectomy did not lead to a steady boyfriend, but the following summer she began dating a man she really liked.

> I felt like I wanted to get it out of the way as soon as possible, but on the first date you can't just slip it into the conversation, "Blah, blah, blah, I've had breast cancer, blah, blah blah."

When her boyfriend invited Karen away for a weekend, she knew she had to tell him.

> We were at his house, sitting on the couch, and I can remember feeling like . . . like *dying*, because I knew I was going to have to tell him. I was sitting, very tense, and I said I had something to tell him. I had had breast cancer, but I was fine. And he was great! He was wonderful as far as dealing with it! If I would have had a negative experience, my whole attitude would probably be different. But I've been amazed. I've had other relationships since then, and everyone has handled it really well.

Although Karen's experience with men's reactions had been very positive, she still has some difficulty in deciding at what point to tell them.

> It's often hard to know when to do it, but my own thing is that I feel like I have to tell them sooner than later. If I start going out with someone on a semiregular basis, and I think that we're going to go on seeing each other and it may lead to an intimate relationship, and also before I get to like them too much, before I feel like I'm getting really emotionally involved with them, I want to tell them because I want to know if they're going to be able to deal with it. If they can't handle it, I'd rather have them out of my life sooner than later, even though it's going to hurt. I'd rather not become too involved and then be really hurt. Every time I have to tell a man I've had breast cancer, though, I'm still waiting [for a negative reaction]—perhaps I'm using it as some sort of test.

In retrospect, Karen feels that perhaps it is too much to expect men to reactive positively on first hearing about her cancer.

> When you tell someone about having had breast cancer and expect him to act really well right away—that is not really fair. Now I see that people need time. Their initial reaction may be negative, but when you get to know them better,

you may find out they're a wonderful person. You need to give people a second chance. You can't just expect men to be like—"Okay, that's fine. No big deal"—because it is a shock to them. Anyone would need time to adjust to that kind of news.

Karen continues to have an active sex life.

It's always interesting to see how somebody's going to react to my body. Are they going to touch it (the implant)? Even though I don't have normal sensation, I can still feel pressure around the edges. The nipple doesn't get erect or anything like that. My reconstructed breast is firmer than my normal breast, and it has a tendency not to be as warm.

Karen would like to get married one day, but she is concerned about having her own children.

The doctors just don't know what to advise about pregnancy after breast cancer. There really aren't any studies on whether it increases your chances of recurrence. But knowing what pregnancy does to the hormones, and the possibility of any dormant cancer cells that may be lying around—that is scary to me.

Nor is Karen sure that she could conceive if she wanted to, because the chemotherapy "messed up" her periods for a while, and now her doctors are not sure if she is ovulating. Although at age 28 Karen says that having her own children was very important, now, in her mid-30s, she finds other possibilities acceptable.

I still do want children, but that doesn't mean they have to be biological children. It could be adoption. I don't see that as being negative anymore. Or I might marry a man who already has children and doesn't want more children. I've just grown a lot and matured a lot, and I've looked at relationships too. So I just don't think that having children necessarily makes or breaks a relationship. Or even that you necessarily have to have children.

Karen has not had a recurrence 6½ years after her diagnosis, although she has had some scares.

Sometimes you get certain aches, something hurts, or whatever. And you get little twinges that you ask, is this cancer? Some of my friends joke—"You've had cancer in every bone in your body." One time I had a chest x-ray, and they thought they saw something on it. They had to take it over again, and then I had to wait 24 hours to get the results. I knew what lung cancer meant, and that's certainly not a good prognosis. I had to wait for 24 hours to find out it was nothing, and that was a terrible time.

In her adjustment, she feels that having cancer was more difficult to cope with than the loss of the breast.

The thing that bothered me the most was not having a mastectomy itself. It was the idea of cancer. I wish I could just get rid of my breast and have reconstruction, but not have cancer. Life was more important than the idea of losing a breast.

In her work as a speech therapist, Karen believes that her experience with breast cancer has made her more empathic to her patients because she knows "what it's like to feel really crappy after chemotherapy." Karen understands that "people need rests; some days they feel lousy and really can't work to the maximum." As a result of her own experience with a mastectomy and chemotherapy she has a "much better sense of when to back off and when to not push patients so hard."

About 2 years following her mastectomy, Karen made a job change from practicing speech therapy to teaching it.

> Cancer put a different focus on my life. . . . I realized that when I was going to school, I was pushing myself to sort of get finished with my masters, and I realized that life's too short, you've got to stop and smell the roses, so to speak. At times I've fallen back into the old patterns, not taking enough time for me. But I try not to be pushed into certain avenues that I really don't want to be in . . . and that was one reason I think that I made the change from the hospital to the school. Even before I finished my masters, I went into teaching full-time. I was getting frustrated at some of the things that the hospital was doing, and I realized I needed a change. The cancer gave me the courage to make the change. The move here allows me a lot more freedom, and it's allowed me to get more involved with the Cancer Society and to branch out in other ways. . . . I've gotten very involved in the Cancer Society. I like helping other people become more knowledgeable about breast cancer—especially about the real practical stuff. I feel very comfortable talking to women in Reach to Recovery, telling them everything they want to know. I've told many people, I've shown friends my scars, let them feel the prosthesis, because I know people are curious. If you get your questions answered, you can deal with things a whole lot easier.

Karen also gives talks on breast cancer in her community and in the professional schools. One issue for her is how much of her own experience to reveal. She has since learned the following.

> It's all in how you present it. At first, I wasn't sure what the audience's reaction would be. But they were fine. I learned to present it as a fact. Not that it's "poor me," looking for sympathy from you, but that I'm just giving you information, and women do have normal lives after breast cancer.

CASE 3: INGRID

Ingrid, a 28-year-old woman, is one of five children, all living close to the home of her parents. She had been married for 8 years and enjoyed her job as a health educator. One of her job responsibilities involved teaching women how to do breast self-examinations, and in the course of one of the demonstrations, she discovered a lump in her own breast. This did not alarm her, because she had a history of fibrocystic disease.

> When I was 16 years old and again when I was 17, I had lumps removed from my breasts, and they were benign. So this time, the doctor just thought that it was another fibrocystic lump, but it happened that this one was very painful for me, and I knew that it was different. It was a hard lump. I almost felt like I could just make an incision in my skin and actually pull it out. It was the size of a lima bean.
>
> The doctor didn't think anything of it because of my history, but he told me to see a surgeon after Christmas. The surgeon didn't think anything of it either, but he did a biopsy and everyone, including myself, was completely shocked that it was malignant. It just blew my mind. I was devastated. I just felt right away, right then and there, that I was going to die. I just saw death all around me. And that really blew my mind for a while. I just could not envision myself with breast cancer. When he said the words "breast cancer," it was like my whole life just stopped. I couldn't hear anything else that he was saying. I just thought of death.

Ingrid had a lumpectomy about 2 weeks later. Her lymph nodes were all negative, and she then had a course of radiation for 10 weeks with no problems.

> The lumpectomy was fine. As a matter of fact, you can't even see where the incision was. The first day of the radiation, they marked me with a dye. They look like little green moles, but they go all the way around. The first day, when they put the tatoos on, it took 2 hours. The tatoos will be on for life. After that, it only took 15 minutes. I felt fine the whole time, but at the very end, I knew I couldn't take any more because it just makes you *so tired.*

Ingrid is also left with lymphedema (an accumulation of fluid) in her arm. She has a pump and a sleeve, which she uses to relieve the fluid. "It doesn't really work. I can't find a way to get it down. That's one of the complications, I guess."

To cope with all of this, Ingrid leaned on her family and her faith.

> I had a very supportive husband. He talked to me, and he just stuck by me. My parents and my brothers and sisters—we are a very close family—they just helped me through it. We all stuck together. My mother is a very strong woman. I never really saw her break down and cry or anything, but I know she must have been devastated. Same with my father. He doesn't say much, but I can just tell by his reaction that he was very hurt. He was very worried about me. They were always around me, asking me how I felt. They catered to me all the time. They were like smothering me. Sometimes I needed air. Sometimes it was nice, but sometimes, it was too much. But I never said "No" to them, because that was their way of showing me that they cared, and that

they were doing something for me. So I just let them be. I just bore with it. If that's the way they dealt with my treatment, that was fine.

Also, I have a strong faith in Jesus Christ. *Really!* That brought me through it. If I didn't have that, I don't know where I would be. I probably would have lost my mind.

Ingrid also received support from her brothers and sisters, and from friends.

I must have touched some lives, because close to 250 people come to visit while I was in the hospital! I never knew so many people really cared about me. It made me feel good. But I don't have that many close friends. It's good to have one person that you can really talk to, who doesn't talk back. Who listens. Who really listens to what you are saying. I did have a real good friend. We went to high school together, and she is the type of person that just sits and listens. If she does say something to me, it's something positive. And she's honest. I mean, you really have to have that. You really do. Because sometimes your mind just goes crazy, and you really have to have a support person. She's a good person. She's been there for everything.

Everyone's comments, however, were not helpful to her.

Some people who are not in your situation say to you, "Oh, I would have done this" or "I would have done that." But they can't say what they would have done, because they never really feel the way that you feel. They don't really know how you feel. It used to bother me, the way people would not listen to me. I would be telling them about my experiences, and they would relate their experiences. I wanted them to understand what I was talking about.

And I think too that sometimes doctors have to be a little more caring, and not just blurt out what you have and then think nothing of it. I'm the happy-go-lucky type of person, and I have a smile on my face all of the time. So they think that I'm fine. But I was *angry* that I had cancer, and I was so young. Why did this happen to me at this point in my life? I was really angry, and I didn't really have anybody to say that to. I think doctors have to be a little bit more sympathetic. Sometimes I just wanted to tell them how I was feeling. My oncologist was great, and my radiologist. I could actually call her on the phone and talk to her, and whatever she was doing, she would just stop.

Like Rosemary, Ingrid's breast cancer experience was complicated by pregnancy.

I had been trying to get pregnant since I was married, and I was beginning to think I wasn't going to be able to have any children. After I started the radiation treatments, I had a feeling in my mind that I might be pregnant, and I had several pregnancy tests, but they kept coming back negative. One day, I just went to my general practitioner, and I said, "Could you please do another test, because I think I'm pregnant." And I was. I was 6 weeks along. But I had to have an abortion, because they had already started the radiation treatment. I had had two doses. So they stopped the radiation, and I had the abortion, and then, maybe 2 days later, I started back [on radiation treatments]. That was hard for me. My husband was very upset about it, because we both wanted children. I did have the option. I could have had the baby and not the radiation treatment. They did give me that option. But at that point in my life, it was more important to do what was best for my health.

Ingrid went to stay with her parents after her surgery, and her parents took her to radiation treatments, along with her husband. After a short time, she went back to her apartment. In 5 months, she returned to work on a part-time basis. Six months after her radiation treatments were completed, a study came out indicating that the survival rates were better for young women if they had chemotherapy. Ingrid was asked if she wanted to have chemotherapy. "I said, 'No.' I was against it. I really did not want to have chemotherapy at that time. But I said that if it should occur again, then I would receive it."

About a year after her initial surgery, however, Ingrid began to have pain in her back.

After you have cancer, you're really aware of your body, and when things aren't right, you have to get it taken care of right then and there. Every little ache that I had, I would always call the doctor. This particular time, I was having pains in my lower back. I was also beginning to feel very sluggish. I didn't know what was going on. I thought it was because I was putting on weight, so my husband and I would jog and do all this exercise. It became worse. It became so I couldn't even walk up the steps without being short of breath.

So I had a chest x-ray, and she [the radiologist] saw two little spots in my lung, the size of pinheads. She thought it might be related to the breast cancer, but I didn't know that at the time. I went through a series of tests, and they all came back negative. But then he [the doctor] called me, and he wanted me to go into the hospital to do some surgery on my lungs. I didn't know what was going on. I really had to pull myself together, because they were talking surgery on my lungs, intensive care, chest tubes. Again, my mind was blown! [At the hospital] the doctors were all coming in, but no one was telling me exactly what they were going to do. They wanted me to sign a [consent form], and I was annoyed because I really hadn't spoken in any detail with any doctor. I didn't sign until I knew exactly what they were going to do.

They were going to do a biopsy of the lung. I did very well in surgery. They were going to remove the cancer, but I had these little cancer pockets all over my lung, so they didn't remove any. They just sewed me back up. Now they're treating it with chemotherapy. They caught it very early, so I have a good chance. I am going to have chemotherapy for about 2 years.

Ingrid is now 6 months into her chemotherapy and is doing well with it.

I'm on 13 days of chemotherapy and 14 days off. It really hasn't bothered me. I really don't get sick from it. It's all a state of mind. I just have a positive attitude that I'm not going to be sick. I'm not going to die. I'm going to take this chemotherapy, and I'm going to be well. I feel great. The only thing the chemotherapy does, sometimes it slows me down.

Since her lung surgery, Ingrid has been living with her parents. Her husband has also moved in with his parents for the time being.

It blew my mind, but it blew his even more. The second time, I was prepared. I didn't get crazy this time. I was more prepared than my husband. He just really thought I was going to die. He's afraid. He's not saying it, but I can tell by the way he's acting. I don't know that he really knows how to deal with it.

It was always just him and me. Each time I was in the hospital, he stayed with me. He didn't go to work or anything. He is very supportive of me. But he is also very dependent on me. I just think I really have him spoiled. He's used to me doing things, like paying the bills and making decisions. Sometimes I felt like I had a child instead of a husband. I love my husband, but I don't know if I really want to be together right now. I really don't. I don't want any responsibility right now. I used to be responsible for *so much.* I feel good not having to worry about anything. I feel free. I just have to think about myself now. I know that's being selfish. I'm not a selfish person, but I just have to take care of myself now.

Ingrid's experience with breast cancer has made her rethink her career.

I don't know that I want to be a health educator anymore. I think I want to do something pleasurable for me. I loved working with people, but I just don't want to work that hard ever again. I want to do something where I'm my own boss, where I can do like I want to. I don't want to be around sick people. Not right now. I've always been interested in art, and I think I want to go to a school for photography. I always wanted to be a camera person for a news station. Or sewing, or design, or something like that. I want to do my own thing.

She has also changed her thinking about adopting a child.

They won't let me try [to get pregnant] again. Because of the chemotherapy. He [the doctor] told me I should have gone into menopause because of the chemo, but I didn't [laughs]. But maybe I will. He said if I did have a baby, it could be deformed. If I don't have children naturally, I think that I would like to adopt. I would like just one. There's something about one, you know? I always said I would never adopt a child. I never wanted to do that. And now it's in my mind all the time. I'll adopt. It doesn't matter.

At this point, Ingrid is starting to do chores around her parent's house, such as doing the dishes, vacuuming, and sweeping the sidewalk. Her mother is still protective of her, but Ingrid says, "I'm a pretty strong person." Asked how her experience has affected her life, Ingrid says the following.

I try not to let anything bother me. I've always been a positive person, but I used to really let things bother me. I used to really ponder and think over everything. I could never make a decision. Now, I don't think twice. I just go ahead and do it! God's given me a second chance in life, so I can't think anything negative. I can't look back. I have to look forward. I really think this situation was a blessing to me, because there were a lot of things that I wasn't doing that I wanted to do. I would put off things, or work instead of doing them. Now, I'm enjoying life to the fullest. I used to be so busy worrying about everybody and everything—taking care of everybody except myself. Denying myself every time. I was the type of person that never said "No." Whatever you asked me, I don't care how taxed I was, "Okay, I'll do it." Never could say "no." Now it just slides off my back. I can say it now and not worry, not feel guilty about it. I don't know if I would be here without that.

It has also caused me to see people in a different light. I used to not feel for people. I think I used to be cold. I never had compassion for people. Now, life is just so beautiful to me! I just feel that everything's going to be fine. I *know* that I'm going to live and be old. Even if it comes again, which I pray every day that it doesn't, I'm going to beat that too. I just feel that. I'm not going to let it get me! I never asked my doctor what my prognosis is. And I think maybe 'cause I don't want to know. I might not even want to believe what they tell me. Now, it's so important to me to just enjoy life. I never really knew just what that meant before, to *really enjoy life!*

THEMES OF WOMEN WITH BREAST CANCER IN YOUNG ADULTHOOD: THE TWENTIES

The cases of Rosemary, Karen, and Ingrid have provided us with a beginning look at the major themes for young women with breast cancer in their 20s. The themes we have identified—achieving of independence, fertility, developing intimate relationships, and developing a place in the adult world—are elaborated in the following sections. These four themes are discussed in terms of their intersection with the breast cancer tasks of adjustment to role shifts, self-absorption, and adaptation to an uncertain future.

Achieving Independence

In the 20s, separation from the family of origin (Gould, 1978; Levinson et al., 1978) is considered an important developmental task. In his study of 500 men and women between the ages of 16 and 50, Roger Gould (1978) describes the major conflict of this first phase of young adulthood as one in which young adults want to become independent of their parents but do not want to "feel the pain of separation." Young adults are uncertain of their ability and right to take care of themselves and, because of this fear, are vulnerable to staying emotionally dependent on their parents. Levinson et al. (1978), based on their study of men's lives, concur with Gould as they believe that to form a basis for living more "genuinely as an adult in the next period" the young adult must remove the family of origin from the center of his or her life.

This separation or independence from the family of origin has both external and internal components. External aspects include moving out of the family's home, becoming less dependent financially, and taking on autonomous roles. Internal aspects include a reduced emotional dependency on parental support and authority. The task of this phase of adult development is not to end one's relationship with her parents but to renegotiate an adult-to-adult relationship. Other studies (Roberts & Newton, 1987; Stewart, 1977) that have focused on womens' lives have corroborated that young women in this early phase of adulthood also work on the tasks of separation from the family of origin. Rosemary, Karen, and Ingrid had physically moved away from their parents at the time of their diagnosis.

Coping with breast cancer, however, involves adjusting to role shifts and a certain amount of dependency. Rosemary, at age 26, relied quite heavily on her mother through the period of her diagnosis and mastectomy. Her mother accompanied her to the biopsy, visited in the hospital, and changed her bandages twice a day in the week following her discharge from the hospital. Rosemary struggled to maintain her independence, however. She decided to return to her own apartment after surgery, instead of going to her mother's house; she pushed herself to learn to change her own bandages, and she drove herself to and from her chemotherapy, despite her fear of needles. She also found the support of other women with breast cancer more important in some ways than that of her family.

In Karen's case, even more evidence of independence is apparent. She didn't involve her mother until after her biopsy. Even then, she waited until her mother wouldn't be alone—showing a "protecting" of her mother—a role reversal. She also acted to keep some distance from her family during the very tense time waiting for her surgery, and tried to get her mother to go out and not spend all her time sitting in Karen's hospital room. Independence was a main theme of her hospitalization. She was eager to get dressed in normal clothes, and to be up and about. She was especially disturbed about not being able to bathe herself or wash her hair.

During her crisis with cancer, her main source of support came from her friends and siblings rather than her parents.

Ingrid, married and living in an apartment with her husband at the time of her diagnosis, left home to stay with her parents after surgery. Both her parents and her husband accompanied Ingrid to her radiation treatments. Ingrid claims that her parents were "always asking her how she felt" and "smothered" her at times. Ingrid's conflict with dependency-independency is revealed in her comment that sometimes the smothering was "nice, but sometimes it was too much." She was unable to tell her parents that it was too much because she believed it was their way of showing they cared, and she didn't want to hurt them. After a short time she returned to live with her husband in their apartment. Following her second bout with cancer (when it had mastasticized to her lung), however, Ingrid separated from her husband and returned home to live with her parents. Although Ingrid's husband was very supportive of her ("each time I was in the hospital he stayed with me—he didn't go to work or anything") he was also dependent on her. She moved home to gain the extra support she needed to take care of herself and to cope with her illness more successfully. She had been involved in a marriage in which she was expending a lot of energy taking care of her husband and decided, "I can't take care of him anymore." Ingrid's parents and siblings provided her with the care and support she felt she needed to get through this difficult time in her life.

Young adults who have only recently achieved independence from the family of origin may have an especially difficult time with the dependency forced on them by illness. Young women may conclude that they have not been successful as adults if they exercise this dependency. Assistance from parents may be viewed as a blow to the pride of young adults coping with cancer (Blumberg, Flaherty, & Lewis, 1982).

The achievement of independence for the young adult may be complicated by the reaction of the patient's mother. It is not uncommon for the mother of a breast cancer patient to feel guilt. Karen's mother said she would rather have had the disease herself than have her daughter have it, almost as if she had made such a choice. As a result, she felt a responsibility and subsequent guilt. This guilt may lead to the mother overprotecting the daughter in the recovery phase (National Cancer Institute, 1984, p. 160). This behavior would conflict very directly with the daughter's need for independence. Mothers of breast cancer patients may need help to work through their own feelings of responsibility to help foster the young adult's sense of independence. It is important to remember that we are focusing here on the first phase of young adulthood. In our interviews with older women, we did not find this pattern. In fact, many midlife women wanted to take on a dependent role, and some were quite angry with mothers who did not provide enough "mothering" during the crisis of illness.

It can be helpful for young adults with breast cancer to have a support system outside of the family of origin on which they can rely when they are coping with breast cancer. This support system can help them to continue to negotiate the task of achieving independence from their family of origin. In the case of Rosemary, she discovered that her involvement in a support group helped her to conquer her depression following breast cancer. Rosemary needed to talk with other women who had experienced breast cancer. Her relationship with her boyfriend was also critical as he "stuck" by her during some difficult emotional times and helped her to negotiate independence from her family. In the case of Karen, although she needed time alone to process what was happening to her, she also relied on a group of close friends to help her sort through what she needed most for herself. Although Ingrid was married at the time of her diagnosis with breast cancer, her parents and siblings remained the major source of support for her as she struggled with a recurrence. One special high school friend, however, helped her get through this difficult time by listening to her. Young women may need to work on building support systems outside the family of origin as they struggle to adapt to breast cancer and achieve independence simultaneously.

Fertility

Although they may not plan on having children anytime soon, young women tend to take their fertility for granted. In fact, it is often seen as an encumbrance, as a sexually active woman often bears the major responsibility for birth control. Fertility is an important component of self-esteem in both men and women. People who find themselves to be infertile experience a real blow to self-esteem and self-confidence. Unfortunately, the literature on life-course development does not deal substantively with the topic of fertility. Perhaps this is due to the use of "male development" as a model for "human development." Clearly, in most of human history and in most cultures throughout the world, a woman's ability to conceive and bear children is of the highest importance. In modern societies, women have fought for recognition of their other abilities, but even today, fertility carries an almost primordial importance. The impact of breast cancer and its treatments on fertility came as a painful shock to the young women in our study.

There are several ways in which breast cancer can impact on fertility. First, as we saw in Rosemary and Ingrid's cases, if a woman is pregnant when the cancer is discovered, abortion may be advised because the recommended treatments (radiation and chemotherapy) can harm the fetus. A woman is put into the painful position of having to choose between battling her cancer or protecting her unborn child. Both Rosemary and Ingrid chose abortion, although this was not an easy decision, especially for Ingrid, whose pregnancy was a long and eagerly awaited event. Having an abortion at the time of treatment means having to cope with yet another loss at a time when a young woman may be overwhelmed with a whole series of losses: loss of health, loss of invulnerability, and (possibly) loss of a breast. A woman who chooses abortion to increase her chances of survival may be left with a powerful sense of guilt. Guilt, however, would probably accompany any of the possible decisions. A woman who decided against treatment runs the risk of having a healthy child, only to leave it motherless. A woman who has treatment and refuses abortion may have to cope with a child who was damaged to preserve the mother's health. All of these outcomes would be extremely difficult to accept.

Future fertility can also be affected by breast cancer. Radiation and chemotherapy treatments can render a woman infertile, or can damage the eggs, reducing the chance of a healthy baby in the future. For example, Ingrid is now thinking about adoption, an idea that she never considered before her cancer. ("Now it's in my mind all the time—I'll adopt—it doesn't matter!) Karen too has decided not to bear children, not because of the damage caused by the treatment, but because she fears that a pregnancy would increase the production of hormones that would stimulate the growth of any remaining cancer. [Although Karen is correct that pregnancy causes biological changes known to favor breast tumor growth, it is also true that research shows that survival and disease-free interval statistics are not changed by subsequent pregnancy (National Cancer Institute, 1984)]. Karen is also aware that the chemotherapy treatments may have made her infertile.

Breast cancer can also affect a woman's plans for future children in that she may worry about the possibility of passing cancer on to her daughters. Rosemary asks, "Do I want to bring someone into the world and have them suffer the way I did?" There is the possibility that a woman who has purposely postponed childbearing (perhaps through abortion) may regret that she did not bear children when she had the opportunity.

Although none of the young women in our case studies had children at the time their cancer was diagnosed, many young women do have children in early adulthood. For these women, a diagnosis of breast cancer may have a different effect. Fran, who was 31 years old at the time of her diagnosis, had married at age 18 and had three children in her early 20s.

Now, after bilateral mastectomies, she reports feeling guilty that she may have passed her cancer on to her children.

> I felt a lot of guilt for that, that I'd put everybody through so much pain and that now my children had a greater risk. Even though I knew I didn't do it on purpose, I still felt a lot of guilt.

One of Fran's coping mechanisms for handling cancer was to think that, "If it has to be you or your children, just be happy it's you. Which was a big help to me. . . . It helped me get through a lot." Fran was also helped with her guilt when she confided her feelings to her father. "Do you blame us that you got cancer?" her father asked "No! Of course not!" she replied. "Then your children won't blame you," he concluded firmly. (Feelings of guilt about passing cancer on or about the possibility of dying before children are grown are explored further in chapter 3.)

In sum, breast cancer treatment can affect a woman's fertility by damaging a fetus, and damaging or destroying a woman's eggs. Future plans for children may also be affected by concerns that cancer may be inherited by offspring or that the mother may not be able to care for her children until they are grown. Thus, the effect of having breast cancer on fertility can be both profound and complex. It is important that young women have an opportunity to mourn for lost fertility, and to work through their thoughts and feelings about future childbearing. For some, the option of adoption may be attractive. Others may decide to forego children because of fears of mortality. For those who would like the opportunity to bear children at some future time, perhaps newer technologies, such as those that remove and preserve healthy eggs, could be carried out before potentially harmful treatments are initiated.* It is important that the issue of female fertility be given more study, in both its medical and psychosocial aspects. It is extremely important and is all too often ignored.

Development of Intimate Relationships

According to Erikson (1980), another major goal of the first phase of young adulthood is the achievement of intimacy. Intimacy reflects "the ability to experience an open, supportive tender relationship without fear of losing one's identity in the process" and of growing close to another person (Newman & Newman, 1987, p. 446). Intimacy implies the capacity for "mutual empathy and mutual regulation of needs"—the capacity to give and receive pleasure. An intimate relationship encourages the dis-

*Thanks to Linda Walker for this suggestion.

closure of personal feelings and the sharing of plans and ideas (Newman & Newman, 1987). It allows two young people to feel meaningful and special to one another. Erikson's theory of intimacy has been confirmed in one study of women aged 18 to 30 (Mercer, Nichols, & Doyle, 1989).

To move toward establishing an intimate relationship, a person's need for personal gratification has to be subordinated (at times) to his or her need for mutual satisfaction. An illness such as breast cancer, which brings with it the need for self-absorption, could make this subordination very difficult. Self-absorption or a withdrawing into the self comes from a fear of establishing a relationship with another person because it threatens one's own sense of identity or from situational factors such as a medical crisis. Because any serious illness involves increased self-absorption (Moos & Tsu, 1977), one of the emotional risks of having a disease like breast cancer at this stage of life is that it may push a young woman toward isolation. A young woman who is not accustomed to being sick suddenly has to monitor her physical well-being, something to which she probably has not given much attention (Blumberg, Flaherty, & Lewis, 1982). This self-monitoring requires emotional energy that may decrease available resources for her investment in an intimate relationship.

Because the achievement of intimacy is a major task, any deforming surgery (like a mastectomy) could make this difficult. With or without surgery, young women may fear rejection and thus hold back from intimate relationships. This fear is tied to the issue of body image and sexuality. If a young woman has not yet formed a committed relationship at the time of her breast cancer, she may come to see herself as unattractive and thus may be unable to take the risks involved in forming an intimate (sexual) relationship. In Karen's case, her initial diagnosis evoked a need to be alone and sort things out by herself (self-absorption). In terms of intimacy, she did not start dating until more than a year after her diagnosis. Her reconstruction has helped her to achieve a positive self-image. She is still struggling with fears of rejection, however.

In Rosemary's case, a period of self-absorption when she was "mean, moody, and selfish" was accepted and understood by her boyfriend. Her relationship was able to withstand this. It took longer, however, for the couple to achieve a good sexual adjustment, because of the switch to a disruptive birth control method. Rosemary and her boyfriend have recently ended their long-term relationship. Rosemary believes it is because her boyfriend wants her to "let go of the breast cancer," and she wants to continue working with breast cancer patients to help them with their adjustment.

In both Karen's and Rosemary's cases, fears of rejection have been unfounded. Karen, who has dated several men since her mastectomy, has been "amazed" at how well men have reacted. Rosemary describes her boyfriend as "very supportive," although now that they have separated she worries that other men might not be. She has heard stories of men who act fine on hearing about the cancer but then never call back.

To spare herself the pain of rejection, Karen tells men as soon as possible, before she starts liking them too much. Although rejection at this early stage could be painful, she feels it would hurt less than waiting until a more substantial relationship developed and then being dropped. Rosemary anticipates using a different strategy, waiting to tell men until she is a long time into a relationship. She feels that, because of AIDS, sexual activity no longer starts early in a relationship. Thus she would have time to establish a solid relationship, sure that the man was interested in her as a person. She reports feeling very good about being told by a male friend, "One boob doesn't make the person, you know. People are still going to like you for who you are. You have nothing to be ashamed of."

Although Ingrid describes her husband as supportive of her through the beginning stages of her diagnosis, she believes that her recurrence "blew his mind." He became very fearful that she was going to die. Because he is so frightened, he has become even more needy and dependent within their relationship. This is more than Ingrid can tolerate at this time, because she needs to take care of herself both physically and emotionally to get well. Here the issue of intimacy and the tasks of a medical crisis like breast cancer intersect in a way to make achievement of this developmental task very difficult. This young husband is distancing himself from his wife because of his fear that she will die, and he will be abandoned. She, by necessity, must become more self-absorbed and interested in meeting her own needs. The capacity to meet each other's needs—one of the hallmarks of an intimate relationship—is nearly impossible.

It is important to remember here that the impact of breast cancer on a relationship is not limited to adapting to the effects of treatment (e.g., mastectomy, lumpectomy, radiation, and chemotherapy). A woman with a history of breast cancer has a higher risk of another bout with breast cancer and may face an earlier death. Also, as discussed in the previous section, her reproductive potential may be affected. The achievement of intimacy, in the form of a long-standing relationship or a marriage for young women with breast cancer represents a major accomplishment. Some may be aided by the tendency of the young to feel invulnerable, feeling certain that recurrences will happen to "other people."

Open communication is a critical factor in achieving intimacy for the young adult breast cancer patient (National Cancer Institute, 1984, p. 144). Unattached single women may benefit from rehearsing what they will say to new partners. Couples may benefit by discussing their concerns and fears, not only about sex but also about the possibility of recurrence and the question of having children. Patients may be more concerned than are their partners, and often need to be reassured that they are loved for themselves, and not just for their appearance or their reproductive potential.

Finding a Place in the Adult World

Levinson et al. (1978) argue that the primary overriding task of the first phase of early adulthood (the 20s) is to "make a place for oneself in the adult world and to create a life structure that will be viable in the world and suitable to the self" (p. 72). Most young adults have a "dream" of the kind of life they want to lead as adults. The dream has the "quality of a vision, an imagined possibility that generates excitement and vitality" (Levinson et al., 1978, p. 91). Adults in their 20s tend to be goal oriented and future oriented—their sense of time is projected forward with an attitude of "everything is possible."

Although the "dream of the kind of life I want to live as an adult" is more relational in quality for women than men, Jenks (1983) found in her research that the dream is very critical to woman as a developmental task in early adulthood. Stewart (1977), in her investigation of the life structures of women, corroborates that women's development during early adulthood is very similar to that of Levinson's description of men's, with separation from parents and the formation of a dream emerging as critical tasks for this period. Roberts and Newton (1987) have since found that the stages for male development described by Levinson et al. (1978) apply equally well to women; however, they did find that women had different ways of working on the tasks, and the outcomes were different. Although many women try to combine career and family in early adulthood, most tend to adopt either a career focus or a family focus. Which route a woman has chosen during her 20s will color her negotiation of this adult phase of development. There is a tendency for a woman to work on the opposite choice later in the life course (Adams, 1984; Stewart, 1977).

Both Rosemary and Karen focused on the career path in their 20s. Both expected that they would marry and have children at some later point. Having breast cancer affected both women's career paths. Rosemary, who thought she would be in insurance forever, found herself wanting to help people after her bout with cancer and now works in a hospital. She is even thinking about becoming a doctor. Karen remained in the same career, completing the masters she was pursuing. She shifted from being a practitioner to a teacher, however, in part to give her more time for herself. Both Rosemary and Karen have made space in their lives for volunteer activities with breast cancer. Rosemary runs a support group, and Karen lectures to health professionals and community groups in addition to her work with Reach to Recovery.

During her 20s, Ingrid focused on both her marriage and her work as a health educator, and had just returned to school to work on her bachelor's degree when she was diagnosed with breast cancer. Since the recurrence of cancer she is seriously rethinking her earlier career choice as a health educator ("I want to do something very pleasurable. I love working with people but I just don't think I want to work that hard ever again"). For Ingrid, art and photography are possibilities for current career choices, having been interested in them since childhood.

Another young woman we interviewed, Fran, focused on developing a family in her 20s. Although she had always wanted to be a nurse, she was working as a salesperson in a department store when her breast cancer was diagnosed.

> I guess for a while—I don't know if it had anything to do with the cancer, or if I would have thought this before, but I found myself saying, "If I could go back and do everything over again, what would I do?" And the one thing I would have done was go to college. So I thought, "I'll just go now."

Fran has begun night school with a career goal of nursing.

With Rosemary, Karen, Ingrid, and Fran, the breast cancer experience brought about a self-assessment that profoundly altered the "dream." Rosemary found that making money wasn't enough. Karen wanted more time to "smell the roses." Ingrid wanted a career that would use her creative potential. Fran wanted to fulfill a life's dream.

Perhaps facing a serious illness forced these young women to reassess their dream with a deeper sense of values. Studies of psychosocial changes in women's lives have found that a major period of transition was most likely to begin between ages 27 and 30. "For many women this time of life was characterized by disruption of one's previous sense of self, altering one's aims and seeking something for self" (Reinke et al., 1985, p. 1359; Roberts & Newton, 1987). With these changes come increased feelings of personal competence and confidence. This psychosocial transition seems to intersect with the reassessment that is often involved as the woman with breast cancer deals with an uncertain future. The result can be a new and more powerful sense of self. Rosemary, Karen, and Ingrid talk about learning how to say "no" to other people. Young women in America are socialized to be "people pleasers" and learning to be more assertive about their own needs represents a moving away from his ideal. Karen tells other women with breast cancer

> to know that they can say, "I don't want to talk bout it now," and it doesn't mean that they're hiding something or can't deal with the issue, but you don't have to tell everybody everything. There's no need to. . . . You don't have to let other people dictate to you.

Both Karen and Rosemary believe their breast cancer experiences helped them learn to set limits and have more control over their lives. Rosemary received validation from people at work who knew her before her surgery that she had changed. Instead of "feeling obligated to do everything for everybody" she picks and chooses what she wants to do. Her colleagues have said to her, "Boy! You're not the Rosemary we used to know when you came in here. You've really, really changed." Rosemary is pleased about the change because she has developed more confidence in herself and in her work. Karen has gained self-confidence as she talks to more and larger groups about breast cancer. "Every good experience is a little plus check," she says. Perhaps getting successfully through a traumatic event (e.g., breast cancer)—"being a survivor" as Rosemary says—strengthens the self-image of these young women and allows them to pursue dreams that they may have felt themselves incapable of before. Also, the fact that young people are still fairly flexible—still trying themselves out in adult roles—may mean that they can actually carry out changes that older women may only wishfully contemplate.

According to Stewart's theory, Rosemary, Karen, and Ingrid, having pursued careers in their 20s, would be expected to shift their focus to marriage and family in their 30s, whereas Fran would be expected to shift from focusing more on her family to a career. In fact, this seems to be the case. Rosemary is contemplating children in the future. Karen also would like to get married and raise children. Ingrid was trying to get pregnant before her cancer was diagnosed. For these women, however, decisions about childbearing were definitely affected by the breast cancer—as discussed in the preceding section on fertility. Fran, who already has children, has had to include in her plans for the future the possibility that she may not always be there for her children, and to learn to deal with her guilt over this, as well as the possibility that her daughters may inherit breast cancer from her.

This discussion suggests that diagnosis of a serious illness like breast cancer can have a profound impact on the young adult's career and family plans. All three of the young women in the case studies made career changes that they attribute to their cancer experience. All three seem to have experienced personal growth, enhanced self-esteem, and increased self-confidence, which have allowed them to make desired changes in their lives. The cancer seems to have imparted a sense of urgency that women usually do not experience until later. "Life is too short to waste time doing things you don't want to do," they seem to be saying. The cancer may change the sense of what are important life goals, from more superficial pursuits to more profound ones. Finally, cancer may make the dream of a career *and* a family more difficult to achieve for those women who have not had children at the time of diagnosis.

SUMMARY

In our case studies of women in their 20s, we discovered that young adults' strong need for independence may conflict with the dependency created by the illness. Young women may conclude that they have not been successful adults if they are dependent. The young woman with breast cancer may need help to cope with ambivalent feelings fostered by the interaction of the illness task of adjusting to a more dependent role and the life phase task of achieving independence. An active support system comprised of close friends, a boyfriend, or a support group can help with this shift in role and the tasks of achieving independence. Although health professionals may judge that having the mother take major responsibility for postoperative care may result in the best medical outcome, this may lead to regression in psychosocial development and to a sense of failure in achieving independence.

Breast cancer can affect a young woman's ability to have children. Women also may fear becoming mothers because they may not be able to raise their children because of possible recurrence and death. This fear, plus the guilt of possibly passing cancer on to her children, also affects women who already have children. Women may need opportunities to mourn for lost fertility, for a fetus that had to be aborted, or for her own children's future. Women also may need help sorting out their thoughts and feelings about future childbearing.

Coping with breast cancer, which brings with it the need for increased self-absorption, can make the achievement of intimacy with another adult, through dating and marriage, very difficult. The patient, by necessity, must become more interested in meeting her own needs, which may interfere with the relationship. Young women are also concerned about how to cope with partners' reactions to breast cancer. Because open communication is a critical factor in achieving intimacy, unattached single women may benefit from rehearsing what they will say to new partners. Couples may benefit from discussing their concerns, not only about sex but also about the possibility of recurrence and the question of future children.

The breast cancer task of coping with an uncertain future intersects with a need to find a place in the adult world. In some cases, breast cancer interfered with the achievement of a dream (e.g., having children) and in other cases the breast cancer experience forced young women to reassess their dreams with a new and deeper sense of values. In their reassessment comes a new and more powerful sense of self, as they learn to be more assertive about their own needs.

The cases discussed in this chapter demonstrate that the life tasks of independence, intimacy, fertility, and pursuit of a dream and the experience of breast cancer can interact in a positive way, promoting personal growth and self-esteem. Breast cancer may challenge independence and may make the achievements of childbearing and intimacy more sticky. Overcoming these obstacles can impart a new self-confidence, however. The earlier goals or dreams of the young woman with breast cancer may be reassessed in light of the cancer experience, leading to less superficial and other-directed life goals. Thus the cancer experience can contribute to the psychosocial development of the young adult woman.

3 Experiencing Breast Cancer in Young Adulthood: The Thirties

In this chapter, the case studies of three women, Dorothy, Ruth, and Laura, are used to illustrate the impact of breast cancer on the lives of women in their 30s. Dorothy, a 34-year-old married physician, was diagnosed with breast cancer when her two children were ages 10 and 6. Dorothy decided on a lumpectomy, but this initial surgery revealed the necessity for a mastectomy, followed 6 months later by a second prophylactic mastectomy and bilateral reconstruction. Ruth, a married psychiatric nurse, with children ages 5 and 8, was 36 years old when her cancer was diagnosed. Following a needle biopsy, Ruth had a modified radical mastectomy and a round of chemotherapy, although there was no lymph node involvement. Ruth also elected breast reconstruction. Laura, age 38 at diagnosis, was single and working as a scientist in a government laboratory in Washington. Laura's surgery revealed positive lymph nodes, requiring a year of two different types of chemotherapy, supplemented by hormone therapy. One year following her first mastectomy, Laura faced a second mastectomy, but this time without chemotherapy.

Dorothy, Ruth, and Laura's stories illustrate the issues identified as most salient for women in their 30s. One of the prominent themes of the 30s is "letting go of the just world idea." Both Dorothy and Ruth struggled to interpret the unfairness and perceived loss of control exacerbated by their experience with breast cancer at this phase of life. Because the late 30s is a time of sexual actualization for many women, "sexuality" emerged as a salient theme for Dorothy, Ruth, and Laura. Dorothy and Ruth's cases provide a look at issues women face in "coping with children," particularly when and how to tell children about their diagnosis. All three women discuss strains in their "relationships with mothers," which are undergoing developmental transitions during the 30s. Finally, during the 30s many women, like Dorothy, Ruth, and Laura, are "evaluating the meaning of work," as they try to balance work with the personal relationships in their lives. In this chapter, these themes (letting go of the just world idea, sexuality, coping with children, changing relationships with mothers, and evaluating the meaning of work) are discussed in relationship to the breast cancer tasks.

CASE 1: DOROTHY

Dorothy, who found out she had breast cancer at the age of 34, is a "modern" young woman, or "superwoman." She is married and has two children, born when she was in her 20s. She also has an MD and has a new job in a health maintenance organization (HMO). Dorothy had begun work on her MD at a prestigious university in New England but had moved to Philadelphia after her internship while her husband attended law school. When his degree was completed, they returned to New England, where she completed her residency.

Dorothy has always had lumpy breasts and had a benign breast lump removed the year she moved back to New England. She had then discovered large lymph nodes in her neck and had those removed too. "I'm sick of all these lumps, to tell you the truth!" she says. When another lump appeared right in the same place as the previous lump, she was not thinking of cancer. Instead, she debated whether to go back to the surgeon to have it removed or not. She knew that if she went in, the surgeon would recommend removing it. "Do you go through life removing one lump every 2 years?" she asks. "There has been a lot written on benign breast disease as a nondisease, so perhaps you shouldn't keep going in there taking out these lumps."

When the lump got large enough that she could see it, she decided to go in. The surgeon suggested waiting a month, certain that the lump was scar tissue around a stitch that had been left in. He was wrong. At the biopsy a month later, it was clear that the lump was malignant. Because of her previous experience with lumps, Dorothy had gone to the biopsy alone. She knew something was wrong when, in the middle of the biopsy, the surgeon asked "What's your husband's phone number?"

Thinking back to her feelings at that time, at first, she remembers feeling grateful to the surgeon for doing the biopsy, because she had been so ambivalent about it. The second feeling was wanting to escape. "I just wanted to get into my car and drive away . . . and then it wouldn't be true anymore." Next came sadness. "I felt sadness—a great deal of it." She also expressed the idea, however, that many of her feelings were hard to put into words . . . "a lot of feelings that I hadn't experienced before."

Following the biopsy, Dorothy spent a lot of time on the telephone, trying to decide what to do. Because of her education and connections, she was able to locate information on the different treatments, plastic surgery, and experimental results. She took a month and finally decided on lumpectomy with radiation. She never got to the radiation, however, because the lumpectomy revealed a lobular carcinoma in situ in the breast in addition to the original lump. Mastectomy was recommended and, because this type also tends to develop in both breasts, a preventative mastectomy of the second breast was discussed. So Dorothy was not really able to rejoice when the surgeon reported that no lymph nodes were involved. What she heard the surgeon say was "mastectomy" and "both breasts."

Dorothy then was faced with another decision. There was no question that the cancerous breast would have to be removed. Should she have the second breast removed, however? She took another month making the decision. Her main concern was her sexual response. "I didn't care how I looked, but I did care about my sexual response." She finally agreed to have the second breast biopsied, and if it was positive, to have bilateral mastectomies. Because the biopsy of the second breast turned out to be negative, the mastectomy was done only on the one side.

Dorothy found, however, that she was no longer able to enjoy her remaining breast after the mastectomy. "The other breast just didn't mean the same thing anymore. It meant cancer." When she found a lump in the remaining breast, she "just sort of got fed up." She was forced again into the decision of whether to biopsy it. She remembers seeing an article in a medical journal that told of a woman who had a mastectomy on one side and then had 19 biopsies on the remaining breast! "And I said 'forget it . . . forget it! I am not doing it! It's coming off!" And so, 6 months later, she had the second mastectomy, this one preventative.

Six months after that, she had reconstruction on both sides. She made this decision because her active life-style made using the prosthesis difficult. This was especially difficult with active water sports, like water skiing and wind surfing. "On several occasions, in front of colleagues from work, I had to choose between pulling them out and appearing flat chested, or risking losing them in the ocean. So, for sports alone, I went through reconstruction."

At first, Dorothy was disappointed with the results of the reconstruction. "I wasn't very happy. They looked funny. They just looked weird. I had hoped it would look better. I didn't look good for about 6 months, and then the breasts started hanging more normally. Now there is some shape. They have some scar tissue and so they're sort of hard, but they don't look like baseballs. They're not perfectly sized. I wish that were different, but . . . you can't have it all." Dorothy also notes that the new breasts are not sensitive. "It sort of feels like I wear armor here." She motions across her chest. "I've got a lot of stiffness and no feeling."

Despite this very real loss of breast sensation, Dorothy does not feel like her sex life has been compromised.

> During sex, my husband didn't know what to do about my breasts and neither did I. During pregnancy and nursing, I found that my breasts were weird. Sometimes I wanted them touched, and sometimes I didn't because they were so sensitive. He would say, "What do you want? Could you please make up your mind so I know what to do [laughs]?" And with this reconstruction, it's sort of the same too. My husband avoided my whole chest area at first, and I just felt that—it's so fake. You know, you're both thinking, "DISEASE, DIS-EASE, DISEASE" the whole time. It's very hard not to think of cancer when you're making love. But I don't much anymore. I mean, it's there and it's quite obvious because my breasts feel different. He didn't want to touch them, because he said, "Well, you don't feel anything, why should I touch them?" And I said "Well . . . [smiling]." So then he started to, and it was good because I was having some reaction, although I can't feel, it's like my brain knows that when his hand is in a certain place, then I feel a certain way, even though I have no feeling. There was some memory—some pathways in my brain that had been gone over so many times that I responded the same way.

Her sexual satisfaction has not decreased, "Nothing's changed, in terms of intensity or anything. They're [the breasts] something that's gone, and [it] would be better if they were there, but it hasn't made our sex life worse."

The change, however, affected her body image.

> I still can't look at myself too long in a dressing room mirror. . . . I'll never forget the first time I saw a nude woman in a movie, I just felt like : . . "Oh, poor Ted! He must be so wishful!" I think a lot of women do feel very apologetic toward their husbands. And I felt it too, that I had done this to him, and his life had been ruined since this has happened to his wife. I don't feel that so much anymore. Now I feel that something happens to all of us. We get gray, or fat, or whatever, you know. We are middle-aged and [we need to] just accept it. If your husband can't accept it, then—Tough luck! There's more change to come.
>
> I certainly haven't hated my body. I have tried to take care of it and so maybe that was part of it. "Wait a minute! I'm taking care of you . . . what's going on here!?! You don't look the way I want you to look!" [Up until now] I have always been able to get what I want out of my body—just by losing a little weight. It's a very subtle thing. You don't look bad. There is nothing about you that looks bad. I mean, we looked that way for 12 years! You look in the mirror, and you don't really objectively look bad, but there is something about it—that I can't put my finger on—that's terrible. It's not how you want to look. It's definitely a control issue. No control over your own health. After all these years of never drinking a Coke, never doing all this bad stuff, and I get cancer. It did me no good.

Dorothy does speculate, however, that perhaps her cancer was due to something she was exposed to as a child, like perhaps "all those bologna sandwiches."

Concerning her marriage, Dorothy reports that everything had not been perfect *before* her illness. "There was, at that time, quite a bit of tension in the family, I think because of the moving back and forth and trying to adapt to people's careers." In fact, she had been trying to get her husband, Ted, to go into marital counseling with her, but he had refused. In a previous illness, he had distanced himself from her. "Now I see that this is sort of his pattern, that when I'm sick he just stays away. He just can't handle it at all." She knew, however, that he was upset when he came over to the surgeon's office after the biopsy, because he had left his lights on in the car and then couldn't start the car to go home! "He was clearly out of it at that point, but I don't know how he felt. He speaks very little about it. You know, he is not at all familiar with expressing his emotions."

One bonus from the breast cancer, for Dorothy, was that after the surgeries, Ted agreed to go into marital counseling.

> It seemed as if the first few months were terribly unsuccessful. Like we were getting nowhere. We weren't fighting . . . it was just a lack of communication. But then something clicked. He's the kind of person who, when his therapist says, "When Dorothy wants to talk about something, then you should," he does it! He's just somehow able to make those changes, and the same with having a breastless wife. I'm sure he would rather have a wife with breasts, but I think he accepts it too. Which surprised me. As a matter of fact, I have found that men who know perfectly well I have no breasts, still come on to me—make advances, and I think, "Don't you know there's nothing there?" I mean, I know there are some men who divorce their wives and marry 19 year olds. They exist, obviously. There are plenty of them out there. But there are also plenty for whom, really, it doesn't matter.

One issue for Dorothy was when and what to tell her children. She decided to be as open as possible. "I didn't hide it from minute one." Later, she says that, when her children ask for reassurance, she does not tell them that she is cured. "Tomorrow, if I am diagnosed with a recurrence, no one is going to say that I lied to the kids," she says with strong conviction. Dorothy tried to help her children to express their feelings about her illness by speaking openly about *her* feelings.

> I've tried to keep my feelings about the cancer right out in the open. Like, say, if I'm bummed out about breast cancer, I would just say "I hate breast cancer!" Or recently, I've said, "I'm going to the doctor's tomorrow for my

checkup, and I'm very nervous about it," and my son says, "Why, Mom, does this mean you're going to die?" and I say, "No. I'm just telling you that I'm nervous." I've tried to open it up, because if parents just talk to one another, when do they [the kids] get to get their feelings out? They can't talk to their peers. So, we talk about it at the dinner table. I want it to be a topic we can talk about. Once, my son told me his science teacher had said something about cancer in class, and he had come home upset. Well, in order for him to be able to talk to me about that, it has to be an open subject.

Dorothy is also preparing her family, in the case of her death.

Recently, my daughter said, "Well, Mom. You're cured from cancer, right? You'll never get it again, right?" Well, I didn't say yes. I said, "No, I'm not necessarily cured. I hope I am." Another time, my son said, "Mom, why do you keep going to these cancer meetings? You don't have cancer anymore." They're always testing me that way. Do you have cancer or are you cured? We have to go through that a lot. . . . The bad part is, maybe I'm trying to leave room for too many possibilities, so they're protected all around. Because my real fears are that if I were to die, my husband is totally incapable of being an emotional center for the family. I know him. He'll just sit in a chair for a year or two. He will. He'll get depressed. And I told him he has got to get married right away, because he is just so susceptible to withdrawing into his own little shell. And I've tried to say to the kids, even though I know it's dangerous ground, that I think people who lose spouses should get remarried, and that if anything ever happened to either Daddy or me, that we would get remarried, because we believe in the family. So that they would accept a new mother, because my husband and the kids really need someone who is emotionally outside [himself or] herself.

Dorothy remembers the first reaction of her son (age 10). He asked, "Well, how do you think I'm going to feel driving to school with a one-breasted mother?" He also refused to come to the hospital because it smelled too much. "But now he will talk to me about it sometimes. He feels he can share things with me." When Dorothy was in the hospital for her operation, her daughter (age 6) "wouldn't get out of the hospital bed." Dorothy says both children were initially very "huggy" and "always want to do 1,000 hugs good-bye."

Dorothy's mother did not live near her, and there had been some shifting in their roles before the cancer was diagnosed. Dorothy felt that her mother got most of her support from her children rather than the other way around. When Dorothy became ill, she found herself trying to help her mother to deal with it. She would try to bring it up in conversations, to give her mother opportunities to talk about it. But "she just hasn't been able to respond to these openings. . . . She's too emotional for it. She just can't talk about it."

I guess I've never been . . . it's strange. You just find out you're a certain way. You never set up your life that way, but somehow that's how it comes out. That really, I just don't know how to get support from other people. [She cries a bit at saying this.] I don't know how to do it. I don't even know what I want. I just would feel too guilty if people would bring me dinner and all that. Someone said to me, "You have to really believe that *you* are the most important person." "No!" "Yes, you are." And I know what she is saying, but I just can't feel it. It's too dangerous.

Since her cancer diagnosis, Dorothy has moved off the fast track in her career, but this has not been easy for her.

During my residency, I was invited to stay on and take a fellowship in a subspecialty. It was a very prestigious thing. But life is too short to be spending all of it in a hospital! I was very upset about whether to do this or not. Because I always like to take the hard way out. Like the guys. So I took a very different decision for me, and it was largely based on the breast cancer thing. Because if someone tells me I have cancer again tomorrow, I do not want to spend the next 2 years of my life in a hospital! I decided to take this job here [HMO], where it's much less tense. And I'm happy. I enjoy what I'm doing. And the cancer gave me the ability to say, "I have to go pick up my kids now, I can't stay late tonight." I just feel like I can say that now. I'm taking the "woman's" way out, I guess. I've got a lot of ambivalence still in that whole area. I haven't completely worked it out, because it's hard to see that you could be in a more stimulating environment like an academic setting, going to meetings all over the world, being asked your opinion, to make speeches, or whatever. But you've got to give something up to do it.

Clearly, this is an area that Dorothy has not completely resolved. She spoke with great enthusiasm about the fellowship she had been offered. It would have demanded something of her, however, that she was not willing to give.

I think women tend to feel that they just want to be recognized by their peers as having done a good job. That's sort of our goal. We don't have the "I want to rule the world" goals so much. It seems to me that feeling you've done a good job is a more worthwhile attitude than trying to rule the world. But on the other hand, if it's holding women back, then we have to modify this approach, which is perhaps too modest. I'm not sure I have the inside self-confidence to really act like a man in my field. I'm sort of uncomfortable with all that. Do I really want to overcome who I am to that degree? It means putting on something else that I'm not sure I want to put on. I mean, I'm in a very good position now. Why drop out? But, you never know what's around the corner. Thirty years from now I could say, "Why'd you drop out?" So I don't want to be stupid. But life wouldn't be so bad dropping out either. A job is a job. I've never tried being a housewife. Maybe I should try that. It doesn't sound so bad right now.

CASE 2: RUTH

Ruth, age 36, was married and had two children, 5 and 8 years old, when she was diagnosed with breast cancer. She also worked full-time as a nurse in a psychiatric hospital. She describes herself as "kind of 'superwomany.' I worked right up until the moment before the kids were born, I swam my half miles when I was 8 months pregnant, I was very physically fit." Ruth did breast self-examinations regularly and "became sort of vaguely aware of this kind of thickening. I was never attuned to thickening as being any kind of symptom of breast cancer. It felt almost like the skin of an orange was under there." Ruth went in to see her doctor, and he said, "Aw, this isn't anything. How much coffee are you drinking?" But he suggested a baseline mammogram, because she had not had one. Several days later, she got a message at work. "Call Dr. P.," and she thought "Oh shit!" "I just knew something was really wrong." And sure enough, Dr. P. said that the mammogram showed calcification through the breast. He suggested a needle biopsy. The day she got the results of the biopsy, she was ready to leave with the family for a visit to her parents in another state. As she had feared, the results were clear: She would have to have a modified radical mastectomy.

Ruth remembers the trip as a "helpful time."

> I really had time to kind of mentally prepare for what I needed to do. I was with my parents, and they were really quite loving. They were very supportive. Their usual mode is to kind of minimize the down side. And I told them, "Look, I just need to feel really down here. So let me feel weepy, and let me be down, because I really need to do that."

One of the feelings that Ruth was dealing with was anger that this was happening to her.

> About 6 months before discovering the lump, I had gotten involved in this wonderful aerobics class, and that was the first time that I had something aside from the job and the kids, that was just for me. I was just rediscovering my body when I had this other, horrible thing to deal with. I mean, it sort of added to my sense of injustice. My indignation about it. That I was just having time for myself, and life was feeling a little more sane, and there was this little vision of a more peaceful existence, when, suddenly, I was confronted with this horrible proposition that I really had no choice about.

Ruth did not try to hide her feelings from her children.

> I was very open right from the beginning. I used the word "cancer." I told them I was scared, and I was sad, and they would see me crying. I would say, "Mommy just needs to cry. She's really sad." I was feeling unable to mother them much. I was just sort of keeping myself going. Before the operation, I

told them what they were going to do in the hospital. I reassured them that I wouldn't be hurt, that I wouldn't have any pain when they did the operation.

The children were not afraid to see her scar after she came home from the hospital. "They were fascinated. My son went to 'Show and Tell' 2 days later, and he was bragging to all the kids about how many stitches I had!"

After the surgery, Ruth demanded to see a Reach to Recovery volunteer.

> I was feeling like nobody was talking to me. And this really amazing woman—she was 72—and she was wonderful! She came sailing in, and I really just needed somebody who'd been through it. There's this universality. Somebody who'd had their breast chopped off, and they could still move their arm and get around, and continue with their life and, you know, be feisty and fiery and energetic!

On the last day of her hospitalization, however, Ruth had bad news. Although there had been no lymph node involvement, the doctor recommended she go through a round of chemotherapy.

> I asked him to be honest with me, and tell me what the side effects would be. So he laid it out, and it sounded just horrible. I had visions of myself weighing 300 pounds, losing all of my hair, sores in my mouth, my menstrual cycle disrupted. I felt overwhelming anxiety. I have a real needle phobia. I hate needles. So the thought of it—to sit there while they would put these needles in my arm—that was as frightening as what it was going to do to me. It's like another insult, just a further horrible insult on top of all this other crap!

At this point, Ruth experienced a panic attack. She decided to ask for some Valium, although she felt this would not be widely accepted by people of her ethnic background. "I was getting into some ethnic stuff. And I had some friends there, and they said, 'Ruth, don't be so stoic! God! Ask for what you need!' So I did, and the Valium was just wonderful!"

Ruth found her major support in this period came from her woman friends.

> I had enormous support from my woman friends. It just startled me, in terms of how supportive they were, and how much that meant to me. Each person had something special to give to me. I just had this real network that I was very dependent on. I needed these fixes from friends—good friends, who really let me be sad. Not friends who tried to cheer me up. People who would just sit with me, and be with me.

During her hospitalization, Ruth's parents came to her home to help out.

> My parents did come up and stay with the kids during my hospitalization. It got sort of complicated, because I felt guilty for their having to do it. And they

would have ways of doing things with the kids that I didn't like. And there was a friction between my husband and my parents. I needed them, but it added to the tension. It was not really free care. There was a price. So I told them I didn't need them anymore when I got home.

Ruth stayed very active through the 6 months of chemotherapy. She played tennis, swam, and did aerobics. As she expected, she lost some of her hair.

I lost a lot of hair. I remember I was taking a shower, and I looked in the drain, and saw this bird's nest of hair. It was awful! I'd look at my scalp and see this sort of shininess. Before starting the treatments, I had cut my hair really short, and got it back to its natural color. And I told my friend to watch me carefully and tell me if I needed a wig. But I never needed it. I would feel sick, too. I would just lie around and cry. Basically, my sexual interest just dropped off. I also went into menopause because of the chemo. That was like one more infuriating, unfair thing. It was one more loss in this whole unbelievable series of losses.

Ruth says that her husband was very kind and gentle, but he wanted to deal with the breast cancer by avoiding it. "I think my husband wasn't available to me then. I was feeling supported, but ultimately realizing it was me that had to deal with it all." Ruth found a support group of women who had had mastectomies. "That was one thing I did for myself." The group was "just a standard support group, but it was nice. A kind of universal experience. I got to see how other people dealt with it. And I guess I felt like I'd handled this pretty well."

The other thing that Ruth "did for herself" was to have breast reconstruction.

After I had the surgery and after the chemo, I said, "I don't ever want to go near another doctor's scalpel again." And for a full year after the surgery, I was totally unambivalent that I never, ever would want to have breast reconstruction. You know, I did the whole prosthesis route. I had the Reach to Recovery sack. Then I got the birdseed—you know—the weighted prosthesis. Then I got my heavy-duty good prosthesis, and that made a big difference. I used that for a long time, and there was a sort of a bonding. I would say to people, "It's like having a baby. You have this bonding with this appendage." But I'd be swimming a lot, and I'd have to shovel this thing around. It was just a real pain in the ass. I was bothered by my asymmetry. I hated it. I would try to avoid looking at myself in the mirror. The kids would see me, and I would feel horrible. I just felt so odd. I felt horrible for me, I felt horrible for them, I felt horrible for my husband. On the anniversary of the surgery, I decided, "I'm living in the 1980s. Why should I not take advantage of this technology?" So I went and saw this plastic surgeon. I had all sorts of anxiety and misgivings. I had a horrible scar and this just really tight skin. And he said, "Yeah. We can do a really nice job here." So I had the reconstruction, and a few months later, I had an areola done from a skin graft on my thigh, and then had part of my other nipple taken off to form a new nipple. The overall effect is wonderful! It's really cosmetically unbelievable! I mean, it's far from perfect. It's not symmetrical, but it's so much better! For me, that was a really important part of the healing. I don't have the same negative body image at all.

Although Ruth is clearly very happy with the results of her reconstruction, there was one unwanted side effect: the loss of sensation in the nipple on her remaining breast. "So, in effect, I lost an erogenous zone. That's something I wasn't told. It's a trade-off." In fact, Ruth's sex life has not returned to normal. "I definitely have a decreased sexual appetite, which bothers me." Ruth does not feel this is because her husband finds her any less attractive. "He's just been very accepting. He's never made me feel that I was odd. He seemed to love me anyway. We've talked about ways to please each other sexually, and he's been very good in terms of his caring and attentiveness."

In considering how her experience with breast cancer has affected her, Ruth says the following.

> I think I'm more in touch with myself, and part of that is I'm kind of at a midlife point of reflectiveness. Dealing with breast cancer added a sense of urgency to all my self-questioning. And I'm still not totally happy with where I am. I still see myself in a state of evolution. I guess I'm feeling some need to do something different at work. But I'm not sure what. So I kind of go back and forth between thinking I need to do more at work, and then I think, "No, I'd rather just go horseback riding." I'm working on all angles of myself— being more playful and really kind of working on having a good time.

Ruth finds positive changes in herself as a result of her experience with breast cancer. She is still exploring, and in the process, she is finding new, unexplored sides of herself. "I have felt that I've really been on a certain journey. I spend my days thinking about it, talking about it." Her "journey," or exploration of herself, is interwoven with her coming to terms with having cancer.

> Oh, it's had a profound impact on me. I am very conscious of having breast cancer. But there are positive things that I think—because I worked at it— have become part of my legacy. At first I was really morbid. I was fighting it, trying to get myself physically back. Manage my anxiety. Then I was grateful for the time I had. Now, I get mad at myself if I don't remain mindful of the fact that I am mortal, and my time is finite. I'm much more selective about what I do and who I do it with. I'm trying to be more protective of my own needs versus the needs of others. I try to go after what I want more. And I'm better at work. If somebody talks about depression or anxiety here, I really know what they are talking about. I also let things go more—the shitwork—I just let it go!

CASE 3: LAURA

Laura is a highly successful scientist, who works in a government laboratory in Washington, DC. Her parents are both quite frail and live in a retirement community in Arizona. At age 38, Laura was single but living with a man she hoped one day to marry. She had just gotten over a bad flu and had a pain in her breast, which she attributed to an enlarged lymph node from the virus. She had her doctor check it, and he sent her for a mammogram. She went quickly through the routine steps—mammogram, needle biopsy, surgical biopsy. Then came the decision: lumpectomy with radiation or mastectomy? "A number of people looked at me, and the consensus was that I was not a candidate for lumpectomy and radiation therapy. I would have to have a modified radical mastectomy and chemotherapy afterward."

In the difficult days before the surgery, Laura looked for support from her lover.

> I was quite frightened. I remember sleeping with the light on for the first two nights. I tried very hard to get comfort from the man I was involved with, but he just didn't know what to do. That precipitated a lot of emotional conflict, because he was neither equipped emotionally, nor was he interested, in trying to comfort me or finding out how. And I was very upset about that. Probably more upset about that than what was going on [the breast cancer].

As the day for the mastectomy approached, Laura began to anticipate the moment when the bandages would come off, and she would be confronted with the loss of her breast.

> I didn't know how I was going to deal with it. I couldn't imagine myself dealing with that surgery. I remember calling the surgeon and telling him that I thought I was going to have a problem, and he said, "Come on in!" He proceeded to show me pictures of what it would look like. Which was a big shock to me, but I think it helped me a lot.

Following her surgery, Laura was visited by a volunteer from the Reach to Recovery program. However, this was not helpful, in part because she could not identify with the woman who visited.

> It was a matronly, elderly woman who came, and I could not identify with her at all. She brought a packet of stuff—some cotton that I could stuff in my bra when I left the hospital—and for some reason, that packet horrified me. It was sort of freaky. It was like, seeing this heavy, matronly woman, that I'd crossed into some other category. It was devastating!

The mastectomy showed positive lymph nodes, and Laura was scheduled for a year of two different types of chemotherapy, supplemented by hormone therapy.

My oncologist came in to tell me all of the side effects. It was hard to adjust to the fact that my hair was going to fall out. I was supposed to gain 15 to 20 pounds. Because of the male hormones, I was supposed to grow facial hair. (I did start to get peach fuzz.) And it is traumatic when your hair falls out in clumps. You see clumps of hair on the pillow, clumps in the shower, hair everywhere! I think it's disturbing because of the implications—like watching your own dismemberment.

Instead of being overwhelmed by these side effects, Laura took it on as a challenge. She refused to let the chemotherapy interfere with her life. In her work, she became superorganized, getting everything done in the weeks before the treatments, so that in case she was not feeling well, her work would not suffer. She would go right from the chemo injections to work. She also continued to exercise, even though her oncologist kept telling her that she would not be able to continue with this activity.

I just took that as a challenge. I also talked to somebody in the social work department before starting chemo, and she said, "Go out and get your hair cut short, and have the hair that is cut off made into a wig, and then you can wear your own hair, and it'll look like you just have a short haircut." So I did. It freaked me out to think of wearing a wig. I also listened to the professionals on how to use makeup to disguise the fact that my eyebrows and eyelashes were falling out. I was determined not to gain weight. I was very careful and watched what I was eating. I ended up *losing* 10 pounds. I never looked better!

Throughout her treatments, Laura sustained a fighting attitude, which helped her get through rough times.

I was very very motivated. I really was going to win this battle. And when you succeed in the small everyday obstacles, your own private little sense of victory is positive feedback. You get a very good feeling about how you're moving through this. Like every other aspect of my life, there's a certain strength I get, and motivation, and even a high, by striving. It's a positive feeling.

Laura describes the series of "steps" she took in dealing with the problem of "body image."

First, I would go to the health club late at night when few people were there. I would have to get undressed in the locker room, and at first I would try to do it under cover, in a back corner of the room. Then, I was big and brave, and my next accomplishment was to take a shower. I remember a real exhilaration. How proud I was of myself that I took a shower in the locker room! I chanced someone seeing me. Then I started exercising at normal times. I was really proud that I had the guts to take it to the next stage. Then I began to change in the front of the locker room. I'd think to myself, "Well, if anybody's looking, feeling uncomfortable, I'll just say—'It's all right. Everything's all right.' " One rationale was that I realized that if I had seen more women [with mastectomies] changing in the locker rooms, I wouldn't have had to ask the surgeon to show me pictures. If it [breast cancer] is 10% of women, where are they? I thought my being uninhibited was all right because those women who saw me would see that the fear wasn't there. Maybe it is a good thing. The last step was when I was at a conference, which was near a lake. Some of us were sitting out by the lake after the evening session, and somebody said something about going skinny-dipping. I felt a big lump in my throat. But the very next day, I went out and got a bathing suit. I wear tank suits and I do not wear any prosthesis. I was really scared to do this in front of colleagues, but they were all going swimming, and I took off my shirt and jumped in, and later I got out of the lake normally, not trying to hide, and nobody paid any attention or even noticed. I was on a real high when I came back, because I knew I'd taken just one more little step forward.

Laura's treatment has had a profound effect on her sexuality.

I think the part that I'm saddest about is menopause. My secretions have totally stopped. Everything's extremely tight now. I don't think I could have intercourse. It would be excruciatingly painful. I'm sad about that. I wasn't ready for it. I'm still on an antiestrogen, so there's no way my physicians would give me estrogen to alleviate my symptoms. A part of me is gone forever. I used to enjoy sex very much. I was very active. I don't think I will ever have that again. I don't even begin to hope it's possible. For me, that is a much bigger loss than the breast.

Premature menopause also means the inability to bear a child. Laura expresses some sadness about not having children. "As you get older, you tend to wish you'd had children. That has been my inclination over the years."

Laura's serious relationship did not last.

He eventually said he wanted the relationship over and promptly terminated it. In the middle of my chemotherapy, he just left. Disappeared. I have not heard from him since. He didn't want anybody who had any problems.

So her opportunity to get married and possibly have a child did not turn out as she had hoped. At this point, Laura does not have another relationship, and the breast cancer complicates the picture.

I have not been involved since. I have some interests and some people who have been interested in me, but I keep a distance. I did meet somebody. We first spent some time talking on the phone. Then, we got together and spent a wonderful day together. That caused me some concern. How was I going to tell somebody who hadn't been part of my life and knew nothing about what had happened? I knew that at some point I had to do this. How do you let somebody start to get attached to you, and then just lay this bomb in his lap? In this case, I decided to trust my own instincts, and, when the time was right, I would say something. I kept thinking about what I would say the second time we were together. We spent a lovely afternoon, and by the evening, he was putting his arm around me, and the circumstances became such that I knew I had to say something to him, because he was going to discover it himself. And I started to say something . . . and . . . he turned around to face me, and he said, "I know." Then I really began to cry. I had been imagining a split-second look in his eyes that I would find devastating, that would really hurt. I was very touched by the fact that there was another possibility. This was a reaction that never occurred to me. Then he put his arms around me, and I just melted.

Although this relationship did not last, Laura feels that she learned from it. She knows now that when someone loves her, it will not matter about her sexual abilities or her anatomy. "I think that if I were to meet someone who attracted me, and I really became involved with him, probably I wouldn't have any hesitation. But I haven't met anybody yet."

Laura was not able to lean on a supportive husband or lover through this experience. Nor did she have the support of her parents. Both parents were ill. Her father had Alzheimer disease and was severely incapacitated. Her mother had a heart condition and has had to return to Washington for health care several times since Laura's diagnosis of breast cancer.

Neither parent knew anything about this at the time. I knew that my mother couldn't handle my problem, because her main concern was with my father. So I led her to believe I was out of town when I had the surgery. About a month later, I decided to tell her a modified version. I didn't think that I could hide something like a year of chemotherapy from a mother! I told her that they had found a lump, that I had had surgery. I don't think I used the word "cancer." I tried to tell her without using alarming words. I think I said they found a tumor, and they had to take it out, but they got everything. I didn't go into any details or graphics, and she didn't ask. I think because of her own fear. By that time, I was back to exercising, and my arm motions were normal. I had my hair cut into a lovely short hairstyle. I really looked great. This way, she couldn't deny that I was walking around, looking fine. My father knew nothing, because he was so sick that all he could do would be to be frightened. No one else in my family knew. That was an extra incentive to make sure that I always looked fine.

Lacking social support from close family, Laura found ways to support herself.

I needed support because I was frightened. But I had to get it from myself. And I did. I told myself that everything would be all right. Every little step I took gave me more and more confidence. As soon as I began to handle one situation with a little grace, it gave me strength and courage, and that made me better able to handle the next stage with grace. I'm a very strong and independent person.

Laura needed every bit of her strength when she began to experience neurological symptoms in her arm and head. The oncologist put her into the emergency room immediately.

> They were afraid that it was some kind of metastasis. This was the first time that I felt real fear, because up to then I somehow didn't think it was serious. I thought I was going to make it through fine. I did not suspect that my life was in danger. I understood intellectually, but not in the pit of my stomach. But in the emergency room this time, I remember going in for the computed axial tomographic (CAT) scan and just shaking. I had never before found myself physically shaking, and that could only be because I was absolutely terrified. I could not stop the violent shaking, and they could hardly give me the injection of the dye for the scan. After many days of testing it turned out to be a problem unrelated to the breast cancer. However, while I was in the hospital, they also took another mammogram and found something that looked suspicious. There was another tumor there, unrelated to the first. So 2 days later I had a second mastectomy. My fear had subsided by then because they had done all these tests and didn't find anything. So by the time they found the second tumor, I was almost relieved. I'd already mentally been through the worst scenario. With the second mastectomy, there were no lymph nodes, so I didn't need any chemotherapy. It didn't take me long to recover. I was out in a week, and chairing a conference in Los Angeles 10 days later!
>
> I didn't stop doing the things I loved. That helps to short-circuit despair. If I were to focus on my mortality and vulnerability, I would never step outside of my house. Focusing on oneself is very detrimental. It impedes one's moving through life with any kind of grace. The best way to give to your friends is not to be unduly cheerful, not to deny that you're ill, but to just be graceful. Almost everybody responds to that.

Laura has not changed her career plans, or changed direction in life as a result of her cancer. She does feel that the cancer has had a positive effect on her. "It showed me I can do a lot and succeed against all odds." She also feels that she "lives life more fully" and "is more sensitive to human interactions, to the good things about people, their kindnesses, the small, subtle ways people reach out, and respond to each other's needs." For Laura, cancer has been a challenge, which she has tried to meet and master, with her own sense of style—with "grace."

THEMES OF WOMEN WITH BREAST CANCER IN YOUNG ADULTHOOD: THE THIRTIES

Throught the voices of Dorothy, Ruth, and Laura, we hear a beginning discussion of some of the issues facing women in their 30s with breast cancer. These issues are further developed in the ensuing discussion of

letting go of the just world idea, "sexuality," coping with children, relationships with mothers, and evaluating the meaning of work. Throughout
this section these life-cycle issues are discussed as they impact on the breast
cancer tasks of coping with anger, self-absorption, adjusting to role shifts,
maintaining satisfactory sexual relationships, and dealing with an uncertain future. In addition to the three case studies (Dorothy, Ruth, and
Laura), quotations from other women we interviewed who were diagnosed in their 30s are used to elaborate these themes. Quoted are Toni
(age 31), Roberta (age 31), Brenda (age 32), Kate (age 32), Nancy (age
36), Lisa (age 37), Sally (age 37), Lily (age 37), Anne (age 37), Wendy (age
38), Pamela (age 39), and Debra (age 39).

Letting Go of the Just World Idea

In the 30s, young adults begin to challenge the assumption that "rewards
will come automatically if we do what we are supposed to do." Previously,
they have assumed that life should be painless. "If there is pain, either it is
unfair or something is wrong with us" (Gould, 1978, p. 168). Because
people in their 30s are already struggling with this issue, the experience
of breast cancer can bring the wish to believe in a just world into sharp
focus.

With a just world view, when something bad happens, it has to be
interpreted as due to something "bad" that was done. In the case of breast
cancer, this could be attributed to poor health habits (diet, exercise) or
failure to self-examine the breasts, to have a mammogram, or to report a
lump to the physician. This type of explanation would result in self-blame
and would be uncomfortable for the individual. Another response con-
sistent with the just world view and perhaps more palatable would be to
direct blame toward the physician or those who read the mammogram. For
those in their 30s, however, when life may already be looking less and less
fair, these explanations may seem hollow. After all, breast cancer hardly
seems a "just" punishment for a "sin" like eating junk food or failing to
practice breast self-examination. Letting go of the idea of the just or fair
world—where one can control one's destiny—may be facilitated by the
breast cancer experience. This may be very painful, however, and may
result in a great deal of anger.

Dorothy expresses this when she says, "I've tried to take care of my
body. . . . What's going on here? . . . After all those years of never drinking
a Coke, never doing all this bad stuff, and I get cancer!" Dorothy is both
angry ("What do you mean, the world isn't fair—I have no control," she
seems to be saying) and bewildered ("perhaps it was the bologna sandwiches I ate as a child"). On the one hand, she senses the unfairness, as if

the rules of the game she has been playing all her life have suddenly changed. On the other, she clings to the just world idea—"Maybe I *did* do something that caused this to happen."

Ruth also expresses anger at the unfairness and the perceived loss of control. She uses words and phrases like "my sense of injustice," "indignation," and "I really had no choice." These feelings were common in women in their 30s following the diagnosis of breast cancer. Examples follow.

> It just isn't fair! Here we both were, we had gone through putting my husband through school, and decided to have a family, and things were finally looking good financially, and everything, and then, BAM!
>
> Roberta, age 32

> That's the thing. Why is it me? I mean, there's no history in my family. I mean, shoot! Darn it! Why me? One in 10. Great!
>
> Anne, age 37

> Clinically, I probably should not have breast cancer. Not according to my diet. I breast fed . . . tried to do everything right.
>
> Nancy, age 36

> I was always known by my friends as a health food nut. I was a very careful eater. I haven't eaten bacon in 20 years. I never ate anything like beef. No fat. I exercised. I took walks. We don't have this in the family. Why couldn't it have happened to somebody older? I was just starting life. I kept thinking, it wasn't fair. It just wasn't fair. Nobody ever said that life was going to be fair, but—I really thought it wasn't being fair.
>
> Lily, age 37

These women were especially angry when they had done what they considered appropriate, and the cancer still had not been prevented. After all, they had been "good girls," following the recommendations of the medical community and were now being "punished." Lisa, who was age 37 when breast cancer was diagnosed, is another example. Lisa's mother had had breast cancer, and so Lisa had a baseline mammogram at about age 20. Ten years later, she had a cyst removed, which was benign. Two years later, another benign cyst was removed. Lisa was very careful to examine her breasts monthly and to have every unusual bump checked. She was also getting mammograms every 6 months. So when she felt another lump, she was not alarmed. After all, it was less than 6 months after her last mammogram. On biopsy, however, this lump was found to be malignant. Lisa says the following.

> I was real resentful that the mammogram didn't discover it. If it [the tissue] was so dense, then why didn't somebody say, "This is so dense! Why don't we do something about it!" I had done everything I could have possibly have done to prevent this. Actually, I think my biggest resentment came after it was determined that I had a number of positive nodes.

Lisa directs her anger toward the medical community—toward "somebody" who should have done something to prevent the spread of her cancer.

In Anne's case, the anger is directed inward. Anne had felt a lump in January and had gone right in to see her doctor. He couldn't feel anything but suggested she have a mammogram. The mammogram showed no abnormality. Then, when she could still feel the lump 6 months later, she went to see a surgeon. He concluded that it was probably an infection and tried to get it to drain for about a month. Finally, he suggested a biopsy, which turned out to be malignant. Despite the fact that she followed her doctor's advice, Anne feels guilty.

> I'm very bitter about that first mammogram I had. I will tell my husband, if I ever die over this, I want you to have somebody look at that first mammogram—check it out and tell me if they didn't miss something. Because I felt it! I kick myself and feel guilty over that. I hate to tell that story because I feel like such a *jerk!* Like [said mimicking the voice of a disparaging gossip] "God, doesn't she know you're supposed to have these things checked? She let it go so far she couldn't get a lumpectomy. She let it go and go and look what happened! She had to have all that chemotherapy and a mastectomy and radiation too. Wow! She must not be very bright."

Anne feels guilty, even though she did what she was supposed to do. It seems that she cannot let go of the just world concept. Therefore, she must have been at fault. She feels blamed—and guilty—in the eyes of the world.

Encountering evidence of "unfairness" creates anger in these women. Anger is not a comfortable emotion for women, however. In our culture, women are socialized not to acknowledge or express anger (Lerner, 1985). It is "unfeminine." One way to deal with the felt anger that does not risk the "unfeminine" label is to turn the anger inward—as Anne does. ("I kick myself.") Unfortunately, anger turned against the self is harmful, resulting in painful depression. It is probably more helpful for women to express their anger in a "safe" environment—perhaps a support group or an individual therapy session. Once the anger has been expressed, women can begin to develop an acceptance of a world that is not necessarily fair—one in which "bad things happen to good people." In such a world, it is not necessary to find a target for blame.

This resolution is difficult, because it can leave a woman feeling unprotected. Brenda (age 32) expresses the following.

> It [cancer] made me feel a lot more vulnerable in all areas of my life. I was pretty reckless when I was younger. I was athletic. I could do whatever I wanted to do. I went from that to being very physically insecure and emotionally insecure. I became much less of a risktaker.

Because the 30s is a time of life when many people are struggling to interpret "unfairness," the experience with breast cancer can help an individual to develop a new view of the world that is more functional for dealing with the later phases of life. As Brenda says, "One of the difficult things we do in adulthood is to be confronted with the fact that we're not invincible, and that came a lot earlier for me than it did for other people. I felt like I went from age 32 to age 42 in a matter of 4 or 5 months."

Sexuality

A woman's sexuality tends to peak much later then does a man's. Men reach a sexual peak before the age of 20, whereas many women do not come into their own sexually until the 30s (Sheehy, 1976; Starr & Weiner, 1981). The late 30s can be a time of real sexual actualization for many women. "There is evidence that many women are able to free themselves from cultural inhibitions and from the demands of childrearing by their later thirties, at a time when their biological capacity for sexual response is still high (and in some respects higher than in youth), allowing a 'late bloom' of sexual desire" (Schaie & Willis, 1986 p. 181).

Breast cancer and its treatments can have a profound negative impact on sexual development and its expression. As we might expect, younger women are most likely to report that mastectomy had a negative impact on their sex life (Jamison et al., 1978). In Dorothy's case, the loss of her breasts was experienced as the loss of an erogenous zone. For this reason, she tried to preserve her second breast. The cancer alone, however, had changed her feeling about her remaining breast. ("You're both thinking 'DISEASE, DISEASE, DISEASE' all the time.") Although Dorothy has had bilateral mastectomies and has no feeling in the chest area ("It feels like I'm wearing armor"), she still gets some pleasure from having her reconstructed breasts touched.

Ruth had a mastectomy followed by chemotherapy and, like Dorothy, had reconstruction. Ruth's reconstruction, however, involved transferring part of the nipple on her remaining breast to the artificial breast. This resulted in a loss of sensation in the natural breast. Thus, she lost an erogenous zone. Ruth has experienced a loss of sexual appetite, and her sex life has not returned to normal.

Laura's case is even more extreme. Like Ruth, her chemotherapy catapulted her into menopause. Even more devastating, the antiestrogen drugs she takes have dried up her vaginal secretions. ("Intercourse would be excruciatingly painful now.") She feels that the loss of sexuality is a bigger loss than the loss of the breasts.

In all three cases discussed here, sexuality has been compromised by breast cancer treatment. The severer the treatment, the more sexuality is compromised. Thus we would expect the impact of lumpectomy-radiation to be the least devastating treatment, followed by mastectomy, bilateral mastectomies, chemotherapy, and hormone therapy. Reconstruction, which appears to have a very positive impact on body image, can enhance sexual pleasure, as in Dorothy's case, or interfere with it, as in Ruth's.

Several women in our sample were able to return to a normal sex life. One important factor may be timing. Consider the case of Toni, who was 31 years old at the time of her diagnosis.

> I hadn't been out of the hospital [for bilateral mastectomies] a week before we had sex, and I thought it would be months—maybe years [laughs]! I don't know if he [the husband] thought it would make me feel better, or if it was something he needed, but we did it. It was such a strange feeling, because you kind of get into a routine, and that routine was messed up. But it's all right now. You adjust. It's probably as good now as it was before.

Compare this to Sally, 37 years old, who, like Toni, is married and has children.

> We don't really have much of a sex life. I've never really talked to anybody about this. I think it's that we're out of the habit. That whole year [of treatments: two mastectomies and chemotherapy] I didn't feel like having sex. Now our son just comes in and crawls into our bed whenever he wants to. I really don't have that much of a sex drive anymore.

A major difference between the two cases is that Sally had chemotherapy. The drugs used in chemotherapy can dry the vaginal tissues. The fatigue common in patients in chemotherapy can also reduce sexual energy. Also, psychological reactions, like anxiety and depression, can interfere with sexual drive. Although those changes are time limited, they may serve to get a couple out of the habit of sex. In this situation, getting a sexual relationship going again may be difficult. Women have often been socialized to feel that the initiation of sex is not "ladylike." Thus they may be uncomfortable letting husbands know that they would like to reestablish sexual intimacy. They might also fear rejection if they feel that they are no longer sexually attractive to their partners (National Cancer Institute, 1984). Unfortunately, the time when women may benefit from help with these issues (after chemotherapy) is a time when connections to the health system are becoming less and less frequent.

Another important factor for women in their 30s is whether they are married. In Laura's case, we saw an example of a single woman in a relationship that did not survive the breast cancer. The single woman who is not already in a relationship and who wants to develop and express her sexuality faces the difficult prospect of telling new partners that she has had breast cancer—especially if a mastectomy is involved. ("You can't just say, 'Hello, my name is Laura and I have breast cancer!' ") Conversely, the single woman does not have to overcome poor communication patterns that have been building for years. She has a chance to start over and to select the kind of partner who *can* "deal with problems."

Although sexuality is important for all women, it is especially important in the 30s, when many women reach their sexual peak. Women and their partners need to learn new ways to enhance sexual pleasure despite the losses they have experienced.

Coping with Children

Many women in their 30s are active mothers whose children are not yet grown. If they had children early, they may have teenaged children; if their children were born later, they may be mothering very young or school-aged children. Breast cancer interferes with the tasks of mothering in many ways. Because, like any serious illness, breast cancer results in self-absorption, a woman is less able to be there for her children (Lichtman et al., 1984). The emotional reactions of anger, anxiety, and depression may also make her less available to them. Treatments may take her away from the home (e.g., surgery) and may exhaust her (e.g., chemotherapy or radiation) so that she is less able to care for them. In a more basic sense, breast cancer represents a failure of motherhood in that she cannot protect her children from one of life's great tragedies—the death of a mother.

One issue for women is how much to tell the children and how to frame it. Some women feel they can protect their children by not telling them or by minimizing the meaning of the disease. Not telling may be an especially comfortable solution for women who are using denial themselves in coping with their breast cancer. "If the children don't know, then it didn't happen." It may also protect them from the pain of seeing their children hurt and from any angry responses the children may direct toward them. One example is Anne's approach.

> No. We didn't tell them. Let's see, one was 6 and one was 3. My oldest one is very sensitive. I don't know, I sort of could have told them, but my husband was like, "Why burden them at 6 years old? And the 3 year old is not going to understand it anyway." So we just didn't tell them. I just lock the door now when I'm taking a shower [laughs].

One woman we interviewed, Kate, made a similar decision. At age 32, her children were 4 and 8. Kate is now in her 50s and regrets the decision not to tell the children about her breast cancer.

> The kids didn't know, but they knew something was wrong, because when my husband called, my mother was crying. My 4-year-old son told my neighbor the next day, "I don't think Mommy is coming home, because my Nana is crying. Mommy's not going to come home." So they knew something wasn't right. I wanted to tell the boys, and my husband didn't. And before we resolved that, we had gotten involved with my mother's health problems. It just never was the right time to tell them. When the older son was 16, he burst out in anger one day at his father, "I know how strong Mommy is. You don't have to tell me. I *know* what she's been through. I know it all!" Apparently he had listened in on adult conversations when we thought he was asleep.
>
> He had secretly known from the beginning! And I felt so bad when I learned that, because my husband and I weren't able to help him with his feelings, because we thought we were protecting him by not telling him. And yet he knew, and I don't think that is right. If anybody ever has anything again, I would not want it to be hidden. Because, essentially, I was doing the same thing that had been done to me as a child when my grandfather had cancer. Whispering, with only the adults knowing. And I did it to my own children, by not telling them and not being open about it.

In Kate's case, it was clear that the fears of her children were worse than was the truth. By not telling them, the parents left them without help in interpreting the dangers and in coping with them. Kate's 4 year old sensed that something was very wrong when he saw his grandmother crying. He concluded that his mother was already dead—a far worse outcome than the true situation. Children who are not told about their parent's illness have been found to experience more regressive behavior than those who are told as much as they can understand (National Cancer Foundation, 1977).

Dorothy took a different approach. She was very open and truthful with her children. She expressed her feelings openly and helped them to express theirs. Like Anne and Kate, Dorothy was trying to protect her children, but she did this by trying to model for them how to handle serious disease and by trying to prepare a healthy environment for them in the event of her death. ("I told him [the husband] he was to get remarried right away. . . . I told them [the kids] that people who lose spouses should get remarried, so that they would accept a new mother.") No doubt, this was a very painful thing for Dorothy to do, because it meant looking squarely at the possibility of an early death. It also denies the "cheerful optimism" that is encouraged by our society in the face of serious illness.

In being open and honest with her children, Dorothy also left herself unprotected from the pain of their reactions. Her older son's angry outburst and her younger child's clinging made her aware how her illness had hurt them. Because Dorothy has not completely let go of the just world concept, she may feel that she is responsible for hurting them. When she refuses to reassure them that her cancer is "cured," she admits to them her inability to protect them (or herself) from the bad things in life. Because parents seem omnipotent to young children, this level of honesty may be frightening to them. Whatever the outcome for the children, it is clear that Dorothy has gained confidence and self-esteem for being able to be so straightforward and honest with her children. Her comment that "no one is going to say that I lied to the kids" illustrates how important this is to her.

Ruth also chose to be open with her children about her cancer. Ruth focused on the mastectomy, however, reassuring her children that the operation would not be painful, rather than focusing on the threat of her mortality. Ruth's solution seems to be a compromise between Anne's and Dorothy's: She was open about what she was experiencing but protected them from the meaning of the disease. Wendy (age 38), who also minimized the disease, had an 11-year-old daughter at the time of her diagnosis.

> I'm very close to my daughter, but she wasn't attuned to how serious it was. In the hospital, she preferred to go to the snack bar. We had tried to make light of it—you know, "Everything's fine!" And she reacted like, "Well, Mom says everything is OK, so why should I worry about it anymore?"

In dealing with children, an important factor is their age. When children are very young, telling them may not be the most critical issue. Lisa, whose son was only 2 years old, says that "it slid right off his back." The main concern for these mothers is the welfare of the children if they should die. They also often feel guilty about how their absence and self-absorption may have affected the child. Lisa says, "I wonder if his difficult adjustment to nursery school was due to my breast cancer." She feels that perhaps she has held him back developmentally. This causes guilt for any mother, because it is the cultural expectation of mothers that they will do the opposite—that is, support and nurture their children.

One woman in her 30s with a 1-year-old daughter, took her daughter to stay with her parents from the time of the original discovery of the lump until after the mastectomy.

> I had read so many times how, if you're going to leave your baby, you should not do it until they're 18 months old. But I had to do it. I couldn't care for myself and her too. She needed a lot, and I was just too emotional. Even when I did visit her, I wasn't sure I was there. I could still only concentrate on myself.

Here, we see the self-absorption common in the period immediately following diagnosis interfering with the demands of the mother role. Her daughter adjusted well to the arrangement, however.

> She took a picture of the three of us [mother, father, and herself] with her, and every morning she would look at the picture and say, "Daddy's at work, Mommy's with the doctor, and I'm here." At first, when she came back, she clung to me a lot. She wouldn't let me out of her sight. When I had enough energy, I gave her a huge birthday party when she was 2. I'll admit, it was a little outrageous, but I decided that she should have this. When I finished the chemotherapy, I told her that I wouldn't be going to the doctors much any more. By this time she was 2½, and she looked at me—"No more doctors?" I said, "No." And she said, "No more sleeping with doctors?" Because every time she'd seen me it was either in the exam room or in a hospital bed [laughs]!

With younger children, the association of cancer with pain and death has not been established, and so they tend to accept their parent's explanations of the disease, and their assurances that "it will be all right."

When children are teenagers, the fear of not being able to raise the children to adulthood is less intense. Wendy, 38 years old at diagnosis, was 42 years old at the time of her interview. "I feel much better now because my children are older. My daughter [age 15] is helping around the house more. I just feel like, if anything happened to me, they're more self-sufficient."

For a teenaged girl whose breasts are just developing, breast cancer in her mother must be especially frightening. An angry, defiant reaction is not surprising. For example, Nancy was diagnosed with breast cancer in her 30s, when her daughter was 15.

> At first, she was kind of clingy, you know, wanting to be with me all the time. But then, her reaction became [that of a] typical teenager. At that age, everything's traumatic anyhow! We took her to the gynecologist, and she [the doctor] showed her how to examine herself. And she came out with the comment that, "Well, this is going to be my fate; you had it, Grandma had it, I'm going to get it" type of attitude. And I just turned around and said "Don't even worry—don't worry about it now." But she does take the attitude that "That's what I'm going to get when I'm that age, so I might as well enjoy myself now." I try to let her know what she can do now to decrease her chances, but her attitude is, "Why not drink soda with caffeine? I might as well live it up!" I think you just have to make them aware, and, eventually, she will know what she has to do to take care of herself.

Pamela (age 39) also tries to protect her teenage daughter.

> She must learn to take care of her body, eat well, and take no unnecessary drugs. It may sound like strange advice from a mother, but I will tell her that

maybe she had better not stay a virgin much after 20, figure out a method of birth control that does not involve hormones, and if she wants a family, try to get it underway by the age of 25.

It is clear that the attempt to protect a teenaged daughter from breast cancer may be very frustrating for a woman and may raise conflicts with other parenting goals. Further discussion of the reactions of teenagers is found in chapter 4.

Of course, not all women in their 30s have children. Laura indicates that she wishes that she had children. In her case, breast cancer has eliminated the possibility of bearing children because her treatment has induced menopause. For Lisa, who had a 2 year old at the time of her diagnosis, the cancer has prevented her from having the second child she had planned.

In sum, several factors seem to contribute to how and what children will be told, including the age of the children, the type of coping mechanisms (e.g., denial) the mother uses, and the communication patterns in the family. We found a range from not telling at all; telling about the disease but minimizing its meaning; to being completely honest, even about the possibility of the mother's death. Each solution has its own costs and benefits, for mother, father, and children. Modeling and role playing could be used to help parents find the right words in advance and to develop healthy responses to the initial reactions of the children.

Women in their 30s fear not being able to care for their children to adulthood and experience some relief as the children get older. Those women who have daughters may feel guilty about the possibility of passing it on to them. This issue may be especially pronounced as the daughters begin to develop breasts. Handling reactions in the daughters (from angry defiance to hypochondria to depression) may be good areas for discussion in support groups, or for individual or family counseling. Finally, women whose opportunities for childbearing are curtailed by breast cancer and its treatments may benefit from grief counseling.

Relationships with Mothers

In the 20s, we saw women turning to their family of origin—to their mothers—for support and nurturance. In the 30s, a different pattern seems to emerge in some cases. The easy return to "childhood" seems to be closed to these women. In her book, *Linked Lives*, Fischer (1986) describes four types of mother-daughter relationships that occur when daughters are in young adulthood. These are (a) pretransitional (responsible mother, dependent daughter); (b) role reversal (responsible daughter, dependent mother); (c) peerlike; and (d) mutual mothering.

In Dorothy's case, we see a relationship that appears to have shifted into role reversal. One result is that Dorothy no longer has enough support. Like many young mothers, she finds herself providing support to everyone else, even when she is ill. She continues to have dependency needs but cannot express them. She experiences real sadness about the loss of the only relationship in her life in which these needs could be safely met.

Brenda provides a different reaction to this mother-daughter situation than Dorothy. Brenda, who was living with her lover at the time she was diagnosed, "let" her mother come for a week ("she needed to take care of me"), but would have preferred just having had her lover and other friends care for her during that time. The time her mother spent with her was full of conflict because

> She [her mother] just felt that she wasn't needed—she thought she'd come out and cook for me, and carry me trays of food in bed and stuff, and I wasn't into that. I wanted to be out and doing things, and I wasn't going to be taken care of. So that was too bad, 'cause she really needed to take care of me.

Although Brenda and her mother had many conflicts during the week, they ended up "compromising," with "me letting her take care of me a little bit, and her letting go of her caretaker role and just enjoying what was going on—neither of us doing it too well." This mother-daughter relationship clearly seems to express some of the strains when the relationship is beginning to move away from a responsible mother-dependent daughter to more of a peer relationship. In a sense, the daughter's experience with breast cancer interacted with this developmental shift in a positive way as they moved toward a "compromise."

Kate (age 32) presents an example of a kind of mutual mothering relationship.

> It was a terrible year. Only 4 months after my first operation [mastectomy], my mother was diagnosed as having Hodgkin disease. It was hard for my father. They had been married a long time. I am an only child. They were devastated from my being diagnosed as having cancer. My father walked around for over a year with a grave face. And everybody was trying to help each other and not let them worry. I didn't want my mother to worry about me. She didn't want me to worry about her. We didn't want my father to worry about the two of us. Everybody was trying to protect everybody.

When Kate became ill, her mother was very supportive, going to the hospital, cheering Kate up, and bringing in a cake to celebrate her anniversary. When her mother became ill, however, Kate behaved like a mother to her own mother—and later, to her father. Kate's father had a very hard time handling the fact that both his wife and daughter had cancer, and Kate became a "sandwich generation" woman, worrying about both her parents and children.

Lisa also found herself unable to get support from her mother. Lisa's mother had had breast cancer herself. When Lisa was in school, she had a cyst removed from her breast. Her cousin (a doctor) told her, "You don't need to tell your mother about this." Lisa says, "And I didn't, because I thought it might upset her too much. Later, I came to resent that. Here my mom was being a mom for everyone else, getting upset for everyone else. . . . I needed her to get upset for me."

In Ruth's case, the strain between her family of origin and family of procreation was too great to allow her to slip back into a dependent role. Although she wanted the type of nurturing her parents could provide, she put the needs of her husband and children ahead of her own and asked her parents to leave. Unlike Dorothy, Ruth was able to receive support from women friends. ("I just had this real network that I was dependent on. I needed these fixes from friends—good friends. . . .")

A somewhat different example is provided by Lily, age 37, who was cared for after her surgery by her husband's mother. She says the following.

> My husband's mother came to stay with us for a while. That was very unpleasant for me, not because I don't like her, but it was a very hard time for me—a very personal time—and I didn't know her that well. I would much rather have had my own mother, but she couldn't do it. So my mother-in-law stayed with me, and that was very stressful. She had so many backward ideas. She treated me like I was at the end of the line.

Perhaps it is only a mother who can nurture a woman in her 30s. In this case, the "help" provided was not truly nurturing and caused more stress then it relieved.

In Laura's case, there was a clear role reversal, with Laura taking care of her mother. Her initial refusal to tell her mother about her cancer reverses the situation discussed in the previous section, where parents withheld the news from their children in order not to burden them. Laura also minimizes the seriousness of the disease when she finally does tell her mother, as some parents do when they tell their children. Like Ruth and Dorothy, Laura needed to find support outside of the mother–daughter relationship. Laura says she was able to generate that support internally. ("I needed support . . . but I had to get that from myself.") She had high self-esteem, built on a life of accomplishment. She was able to "reframe" her cancer experience as a series of accomplishments that contributed further to her self-esteem. She took a great deal of pride in her ability to handle everything independently—perhaps a type of counterdependency.

Fathers are also sometimes involved, especially if the mother is not available, although the patterns of the relationship may be different. Lisa, whose mother had died of breast cancer, was helped by her father following her surgeries. Her father was also providing a more traditional masculine type of help: money. "He's helping us financially. And he paid for our trip to Bermuda last summer. I said, 'Daddy, please do this for me.' And he did." Lisa sees this as a kind of indulgence that he would probably not have provided but for her illness. Here Lisa sounds like a little girl, but in a way girls behave with fathers rather than mothers.

In the 30s, we found strains in the mother–daughter relationship as the relationships shifted away from the "pretransitional" (responsible mother, dependent daughter) relationship. As children settle into adult roles and have children of their own, a period of stability may follow in which "both parents and children remain relatively independent" (Stueve & O'Donnell, 1984). Stueve and O'Donnell (1984) found that women in their 30s were more likely than older women to be preoccupied with establishing their own identities and disengaging from their parents. This preoccupation may be the reason that it was difficult for women with breast cancer to turn to their mothers for help—they believed they should be able to make it without support from their mothers.

In a time of illness, when some regression is common, women find themselves unable to return to their earlier dependent relationship. Some have become mothers themselves and put their caregiving responsibilities ahead of their own need to be nurtured. Others have mothers who are themselves ill and in need of care. One result is that the women who get breast cancer in their 30s seem a lonely group. Children are not old enough to provide support. Husbands seem distant, perhaps focused heavily on their own careers (Levinson et al., 1978) or overwhelmed with the responsibilities of their families' needs and their wives' illnesses. Some women are able to gain support from women friends (e.g., Ruth), but many women in their 30s have been so busy with the dual responsibilities of jobs and families that they have not had time to nurture friendships. Women in their 30s also report feeling isolated in breast cancer support groups because these groups tend to be dominated by midlife women who have a different set of problems. If women in their 30s are visited by a Reach to Recovery volunteer who is an older woman, and if they cannot identify with her, even this minimal support can be lost. Women at this age may need to learn how to ask for support when they need it and how to build support into their lives.

Evaluating the Meaning of Work

Studies of life-course development show that many women start off on one track in their 20s, and then in their thirties they change course and explore the possibilities of the other track (Adams, 1983; Stewart, 1977). If they started with a focus on family and children, they wanted to try themselves out in careers in their thirties. If they started in careers, they wanted to have families in their thirties. This redirection may also involve the discovery of a more creative, impulsive or introspective side of their personalities. Gould (1978) describes the 30s as a time of opening up to what's inside—a time of intense searching about who one really wants to be.

Research on *men* in their 30s shows that this is a time of accomplishment in their careers (Gould, 1978; Levinson et al., 1978). For those in the professions, this is the time when they are working to establish a reputation, make partnership, get tenure, move up the ladder in the corporation. For women, this is a recent opportunity. Even today, most women are not on the same kind of career ladder. Some start out on this ladder, but in the 30s, they begin to hear the biological clock ticking and decide to devote energies to establishing a family. Others try to do both, although this can be very difficult. Still others have traditional families, focusing their energies on their families in their 20s and then developing careers in their 30s as their children are gaining independence.

Both Dorothy and Ruth fall into the category of "superwomen," entering demanding careers at the same time they were establishing their families. Dorothy's experience with breast cancer has contributed to a process of reevaluation. She has tried to succeed in a "man's world" and knows she has the ability to "make it." She is becoming aware of the costs, however. ("You've got to give something up to do it.") By making her aware of her own mortality, breast cancer has forced Dorothy to decide if this is how she really wants to spend her time. She has taken a less demanding job, working in an HMO where she has limited, predictable hours instead of taking a fellowship in a subspecialty in an academic setting, where both demands and opportunities would be greater. She has mixed feelings about this decision, calling it the "woman's position." She sees the demands of success in her field as incompatible with who she is—a woman. The breast cancer provides a legitimate reason for stepping off the fast track. She now does not have to "play the game" if she does not want to. She even contemplates becoming a homemaker, which "doesn't sound so bad right now."

Ruth too finds herself reflecting on how she wants to live her life and how much energy she wants to give to work. Ruth feels that her experience with breast cancer has contributed to this. ("Dealing with breast cancer added a sense of urgency to all my self-questioning.") She vacillates between wanting to "do more" at work, to "do something different at work," and to "just go horseback riding."

Here we see a kind of interaction of a life task and breast cancer. Women in their 30s are already experiencing an "intense searching about who one really wants to be." Breast cancer requires a woman to reconsider the meaning of life. It makes women realize that their lives may be limited, intensifying the need not to waste time. Women who have been struggling to manage demanding careers and raise families may find that breast cancer gives them an excuse to ease up. Perhaps these women, often the first generation of women in their fields, have felt that they had to prove they could make it. They were representing their gender—an enormous burden. Breast cancer gives them a legitimate reason to escape without a sense of failure.

Laura, a scientist, is also in a very demanding career in which she is one of very few women. Although Laura has not questioned her career choice as a result of her experience with breast cancer, she does want to develop the personal side of her life. Up until now, she seems to have followed a male model of development. She never thought at all about marriage or having children in her 20s. Women in traditionally male fields find that they have to work harder, do better, and constantly fight the subtle and not so subtle sexism in the workplace. This makes it difficult to devote time to developing relationships that might lead to intimacy and marriage. By her late 30s Laura has succeeded in her career and would like to find a committed relationship. Her breast cancer interferes, however. She has had two mastectomies and has lost her interest in sex because of the hormonal treatments she takes. Her experience of being left by her boyfriend after becoming ill makes her unsure if she will be able to "meet somebody," although she continues to hope.

In Laura's case, the breast cancer and its treatment seems to interfere with rather than enhance a natural process for the 30s. We would expect a woman in her late 30s who has devoted herself to her career to begin to shift focus and develop the personal side of her life. Breast cancer has made this more difficult for Laura. Laura's response is to treat her cancer as a career goal. She uses the skills she has applied so successfully in her career to cope with her illness.

Another woman we interviewed, Nancy, age 36 at diagnosis, had her first child when she was 17 years of age and now has three teenagers. Unlike Dorothy, Ruth, and Laura, Nancy started out her early adulthood with a focus on family and children, but just before her diagnosis with breast cancer had decided to begin a 4-year college program, leading to a job in physical education. After focusing on family and home during her 20s and early 30s, she had decided to try herself out in a career. Nancy's experience with breast cancer gave her a reason to reevaluate her decision to begin a college education—"Do I want to spend four years as a full-time student, and spend that much time away from my home and my family?" Nancy decided not to pursue a college degree at this point and has been doing volunteer work on physical fitness with chemotherapy patients.

Although she was on a different path than Dorothy, Ruth, and Laura, who had been on the career track before being diagnosed with breast cancer, she too is evaluating the meaning of work.

SUMMARY

according to whom?

From interviews with women in their 30s, it appears that the breast cancer experience intensifies a young woman's struggle to let go of the just world view that is common in this developmental phase. Breast cancer patients need to come to terms with an uncertain future, which means a future that is outside of the control of the patient. The just world view makes this task more difficult to attain. Anger that bad things have happened "when I have tried to do everything right" and guilt that the woman could have prevented her illness were expressed by many of the women we interviewed who were diagnosed in their 30s. Because the 30s is a time when adults are already struggling to interpret "unfairness," the experience with breast cancer can help a woman to let go of the just world idea. Women with breast cancer in their 30s may benefit from ventilating their anger and guilt. They may then be able to develop a new world view in which outcomes are not entirely under individual control.

Although sexuality is important to women of all ages, it is especially important to women in their 30s. Thus, the task of maintaining satisfactory sexual relationships received special emphasis in this life stage. Breast cancer and its treatment made sexual expression more difficult. Women and their partners may need to learn to develop ways to enhance sexual pleasure despite the losses they have experienced. This topic tends to be overlooked by physicians as well as in support services for breast cancer patients.

Many women in their 30s are active mothers with small children or young adolescents. Breast cancer can interfere with mothering tasks in two ways. First, it creates self-absorption, which takes attention away from children. Second, it makes a woman feel that she cannot protect her children, a primary function of mothering. One issue for these women is how and how much to tell their children about their breast cancer. In our study, we found a range of reactions, from not telling them at all; to telling them about the disease but minimizing its importance; to being completely honest, even about the possibility of the mother's death. Women and their husbands may need help in coming to a decision that is best for all members of the family. Women whose childbearing opportunities are curtailed by breast cancer or its treatment may benefit from grief counseling.

In the 30s, we found strains in the mother-daughter relationships, as the daughters believed they should be able to make it without support from their mothers. In a time of illness, when some regression is common, women found themselves unable to return to their earlier dependent relationship with their mothers. In some cases, the adult daughters took care of their mothers emotionally during their illness. Many of these daughters emerge as vulnerable to loneliness—without support in the mother-daughter relationship nor time for nurturing relationships with friends. It seems that women in their 30s have difficulty shifting into the more dependent roles so often necessitated by illness. Women in this age group may need to learn to accept their dependency needs and to build more support into their lives.

Women in their 30s are often focusing on changing direction from that taken in their 20s: Career-oriented women may want to devote more energy to developing relationships, and family-oriented women may want to focus on careers. Breast cancer requires a woman to face an uncertain future. This leads to a reassessment of what is of value in life and how time could best be spent. This coincides with the woman's change in direction during her 30s. It can help a woman get off the fast (career) track without experiencing a sense of failure. It can also complicate a shift to family focus if the treatment has interfered with fertility. For a woman who is seeking fulfillment in a career, it may provide new opportunities, or it may cause her to limit her goals.

4 Experiencing Breast Cancer in Midlife: Part I

The following case studies of Jessica, Beth, and Sandra are examples of how women in midlife experienced breast cancer. Jessica was 45 years old, 3 years into her second marriage, and had one son who was a senior in high school when she was diagnosed with breast cancer. Jessica had a modified radical mastectomy without further treatment and elected breast reconstruction. Beth was 51 years old, married for 30 years, and had five children—the youngest in high school and the oldest married—when she discovered her malignancy. Beth was also working part-time. Beth had a modified radical mastectomy and, after much encouragement from her daughters, decided on breast reconstruction. Sandra, 40 years old, a married suburban homemaker and part-time student with four children, ranging in age from 10 to 20 years, had a modified radical mastectomy following two medical opinions. After several positive lymph nodes were discovered, a course of chemotherapy was recommended. One year following her first mastectomy, Sandra elected to have a prophylactic mastectomy on the second breast, followed by breast reconstruction.

The stories of Jessica, Beth, and Sandra illustrate some of the themes that emerged from our interviews as being most salient for women experiencing breast cancer in midlife. Some breast cancer treatments (e.g., mastectomy) and the task of preserving a satisfactory body image can interact with a midlife concern about "body image" and physical aging in two different ways. Jessica and Beth had difficulty adjusting to an altered body image following their mastectomies—hiding their scars from their husbands for many months. Sandra, having been uncomfortable with her body before surgery, seemed to be more comfortable with and appreciate her body more following her mastectomy. As children grow up and leave the home, one of the tasks confronting a midlife couple is renegotiation of their marital roles. In Sandra's case, communication problems were a major stumbling block in negotiating new marital roles at midlife as well as in integrating the couple's reaction to the breast cancer experience. In Beth and Jessica's cases, a diagnosis of cancer actually strengthened the marital unit by facilitating more intimacy between the marital partners.

The midlife woman is often coping with adolescent children who may have an especially difficult time coping with breast cancer because they are struggling for independence. Jessica's son's preparation for leaving home conflicted with her special needs for closeness and support as she faced a life-threatening illness, whereas Sandra's adolescent son ignored her situation at the time of diagnosis and mastectomy because he was too involved in his own life. In Beth's case her 16-year-old daughter was very concerned but channeled her feelings into school projects.

Following the three case studies, the three themes of body image, marriage, and relationships with adolescent children are discussed as they interact with various aspects of the breast cancer tasks. Additional themes relevant to midlife women are discussed in chapter 5.

CASE 1: JESSICA

Jessica was 45 years old when she found out she had breast cancer. She was 3 years into her second marriage and had one son, who was a senior in high school. Jessica was an only child, whose parents were living. Her first symptom was a stain on her nightgown.

> I had bleeding from the nipple. I thought it was just a little irritation, and I didn't pay too much attention to it. I thought as far as breast cancer was concerned, the indicator was a lump. I must admit I didn't examine myself on a regular basis. I did it occasionally, like most people. My husband said, "I think you'd better see about that." So at my next doctor's visit, I mentioned it along with a few other minor things. The nurse who was interviewing me had a definite reaction to that. As far as she was concerned, the other things were minor. This was of prime importance.
>
> The doctor said he wasn't sure if it was a lump or not. He wanted me to have a mammogram. I have a friend who lives near the doctor's office, and I decided to stop by and see her after the visit. Well, by the time I got over there, this whole thing really did hit me. *This is something to be concerned about!* When I told my friend, she got very upset. She was more upset than I was.

After her mammogram, Jessica's doctor called and told her to see a surgeon. She continued to be calm.

> I just wasn't as alarmed as other people. I don't know if I was just holding my emotions tight or what. I just thought, "It's not going to be cancer." I know a few people who had scares and they were fine. So I thought this was going to

be my case too. I just thought, "This is the thing you do. You get it checked out and then you just go on with your life." I think at the time I was more anxious about finding the right doctor than what was the matter with me.

Jessica had a relative who was a physician, and he recommended that she see an oncologist before going to a surgeon.

> He felt that an oncologist has an expertise and could really give us a picture of what was probably going to be the outcome. This was just exactly the case. It was certainly incredible. He told me pretty much exactly the measurement of the lump, and that it was intraductal. He spent a lot of time with me. He was very considerate. He explained everything, answered all my questions. He was wonderful throughout the whole thing. It made a big difference.

When Jessica did see the surgeon, he biopsied the lump, and found that it was malignant, and that it had spread beyond the duct—"enough to warrant a mastectomy."

> Mentally, I think I accepted it. I knew that at that point, I had to deal with having the surgery. I thought I was doing pretty well, but the Saturday night before the surgery, my husband took me out to a movie. Unfortunately, we went to a movie that was too heavy for me at that moment. We got out of the movie and were driving up the road and I just said to him right out—"I'm not going. I'm not going to the hospital. I'm not going to do this!" I just decided to deny the whole thing and go the other way. Watching that serious movie just brought my emotions right up to the surface, and I was just saying everything that was going through my mind. It was just like purging myself. I guess all these things were just under the surface, and they just came out. Once I got myself together and calmed down, I was pretty much OK.

After the mastectomy (modified radical), Jessica learned that she did not have to have any further treatment. She had no positive lymph nodes.

> The doctor told me, "You are going to go floating out on cloud nine, but the time will come when this really will set in on you, and you will be depressed." It happened to me after a couple of weeks. It was awful weather, and I was by myself a lot of the time. When I was feeling really down, I called the woman who had come to see me in the hospital from Reach to Recovery. I called her twice and left messages, and she never did return my call. That one phone call would have made me feel a little better. I just needed a little bit of encouragement—someone to say, "Yeah, I know." Something like that. I did eventually talk to another woman who had been through a mastectomy, and I said, "It's so strange—when I swallow something cold my whole chest feels cold!" We could share those kinds of experiences. I could say, "Did you find it very painful to do the exercises?" Doctors don't tell you these kinds of things. They don't really know.

Jessica stayed away from work for almost 2 months and didn't really feel back to her usual level of energy for almost 6 months. She attributes this to the effect of the anesthesia. At that time, Jessica went in for reconstruction. She had known she would want it from the beginning.

> It was a goal. It was one of the things that helped keep me going. I think it makes you feel a whole lot better about yourself. Even though the result might not be perfect, it sure is better than having that vacancy there.

Before the reconstruction was completed (an implant with a saline solution was used to stretch the skin before insertion of the implant), however, Jessica went in for a mammogram on the first anniversary of her mastectomy.

> I was feeling wonderful. I thought, "I have had the surgery, I am right in the middle of my reconstruction, I am feeling great." He did the mammogram, and then he wanted to do a sonogram, and I thought, "Something is wrong!" Unfortunately, the radiologist wasn't very kind. He just said, "Well, there is a lump. The surgeon may or may not want to do anything about it." This was probably one of the lowest points for me. Everything was going wonderfully, and then he dumped this on me. And he was very, very abrupt. Very insensitive.

Jessica's surgeon aspirated the lump, and it turned out to be only a cyst. Exactly 1 year later, however, on the second anniversary of her surgery, another lump appeared.

> Then, the following year, I go in and the same thing comes up. And I'm thinking, "This can't be happening!" This time, I had a woman, and she was very sensitive. She explained that the only way to tell if this lump was malignant was by biopsy. So I said, "What about this anesthesia? I just feel so bad afterward. I come out of it so slowly, and it's really hard on me." I just didn't want to really face that. So they did the biopsy with local anesthesia and IV sedation. They took me into the radiology department, and they used ultrasound, or whatever you call it, to locate it [the lump], so he would know where he was going. They were in the process of marking it, and I lost it. I said, "I've got to get out of here!" It felt like a big wave of the ocean coming over me. I just broke out in a cold sweat, and I felt that my head was spinning. I couldn't stand being in there. It was kind of dark and back in the corner. The curtains were drawn. I felt like I was in a hole! I think part of it was that I just didn't know what the IV sedation was going to be like, and part of it was that I didn't want to have another biopsy. But it turned out that I did real well with the local anesthesia. And the biopsy turned out OK too.

At the time of her interview, 3 years after her mastectomy, Jessica is still adjusting to an altered body image.

> I've slowed down since the mastectomy, and I've put on some weight. I'm not as physically active as I used to be. I don't do aerobics anymore. I don't do much in the way of exercise. I never got a prosthesis, because I thought, "If

you're going to have reconstruction, why bother?" So what I did was, I had a padded bra, and I would wear this foam cup [made for putting in bathing suits] inside the padded bra. And I was fairly comfortable. There was some air space, so I was not too hot.

The reconstruction is not perfect, but I can wear a bra, and I feel comfortable and I look pretty good. I have to supplement the shape of my breast in the nipple area, just to make it look good. I never had the nipple reconstruction, because I just didn't feel like going again. By that time, I really had had enough. And I have a real ugly keloid scar from my surgery. I *can* wear a bathing suit. You really can't tell unless you knew and would look. Because, believe me, I'm my own worst critic, and I can stand there and look this way and that way, and I don't think anybody could tell. I feel comfortable to go out on the beach. The only thing I really can't wear is sleeveless clothes, because I have an indentation there.

Jessica feels her mastectomy had a negative effect on her sexual activity.

It probably has had some effect on it [sex life]. At first, I was very conscious of it. Of course, at first, I was very sore. My husband was very attentive, as far as holding me, and cuddling me. He would rub my back. We were very close, but it took a while until we were comfortable with actually having sex. I think he was more afraid of hurting me than I was, but I was a little bit uncomfortable to have him see me the first time. He respected that. He didn't force me to face the fact of him looking at me. He felt that whenever I was ready, that would be okay with him. And that helped. That made it easier.

Then, when I was going through the reconstruction, it was a little hard, because this thing [the implant] was there, and I was afraid not to be careful of it. I didn't want to hurt anything. So our sex wasn't as frequent as it was before. I did withdraw to a certain degree. I think I went through stages of that. Each time I had the possibility of a recurrence, I drew into myself a little bit for a while. Things have gotten to the point where they're improving now.

Jessica's husband was her main source of support throughout the ordeal of her breast cancer. She feels very grateful that her previous marriage had ended in divorce before her diagnosis.

With my previous husband, it was very traumatic. He had the kind of midlife crisis no woman wants to go through—drinking, running around, holding out money—all the worst possible things combined to make you feel degraded, unwanted, and unattractive. He made me feel terrible. [According to him] it was my fault that he drank. Everything he did was my fault. For several years, I had no control over my life, and at one point, I just decided that I was going to have some control. So I started to do some things for myself. I think I just got so angry, to the point that I just decided that I wasn't going to take that any more. It [the separation] was very stressful, but it was also the biggest relief of my life. I learned a lot about myself. I won't ever let anybody control me again like that. *Never!* The same way I won't let a doctor control, or even let cancer control me!

My [current] husband has been very supportive. He did everything he could possibly do, emotionally even more than doing things like cleaning the house up, cooking a meal, or taking me to the doctor. He did all those things, like a lot of men would do, but they wouldn't give you moral support. He did do that. He seems to sense how I feel, and he doesn't let me get too far down. He makes me aware of the fact that I'm doing something that I don't really want to do—let all these things get to me and making things a lot worse than they need to be—making myself more depressed.

I think we have a pretty good relationship. We have a give and take and an understanding. We both are able to say, "I need some support from you. I need you to listen to what I'm saying. Pay a little more attention to what I'm saying. This is really bothering me." As close as our relationship is, and we do have a lot of give and take, we don't always agree on everything, but at least we listen to each other.

Jessica feels that because they have only been married for several years, they are different from other couples their age.

We like to do a lot of things together. I think a lot of people, if they've been married a longer time, do more individual things than we do. For many people, if they didn't have their kids, I don't know what they would talk about. We have a lot more than that going for us.

Jessica was also able to receive support from the I Can Cope program of the local American Cancer Society.

I went to a lot of the lectures. I really think that a support group does a lot of good. It meant a lot to me to get that information and particularly to hear the people talk about their feelings. It helped me to know that I wasn't the only one!

Some of Jessica's friends were supportive, but she is bitter about those who were not.

A few friends did keep in touch with me, but a lot of people didn't, and I was really hurt. I guess it's their protective mechanism not to get too close. They don't know what to say. They don't want to know too much about it. They don't want to think that it can happen to them. I know by the reactions of some people when I see them and talk to them, especially at first, that they didn't want to know. I wouldn't say that they think they can get cancer from me, but they are wary of the situation.

I think you choose some people you are going to share it with, like anything else that is personal. You feel they are going to be receptive, and sometimes they disappoint you. I have one friend that I thought would be right with me. She came over the day after I came home from my biopsy and brought lunch over. But when I had the mastectomy, she never once came to see me, although she lives very near the hospital. She sent flowers. Never once did I see her. Never once did she call me. I really was disappointed. I still am. I still find that I have some resentment toward her. While flowers are nice, when you are close enough to somebody—I mean I have been a real confidant of hers over the years and vice versa. We have known each other on a very personal level. I thought, "As many feelings as we ever shared with each other, even if she had said to me, 'I'm having trouble dealing with this. I hope you will understand. Please try to understand.' " But nothing. I have never really talked to her about this because our friendship at this point is just an occasional contact and nothing more than that.

Nor did Jessica find her mother to be helpful to her. At the time of Jessica's surgery, her mother was herself recovering from a lengthy illness.

She really did try to be supportive of me. She came to see me, and brought me presents and things like that. But as much as I got on a personal level was, "Well, I know how you feel." I'm sure that's very true, but her way of saying it was like, "Now you know how I feel." What she said sounded like it was the reverse of what she really meant. She has a way of turning everything back to herself. I don't know. I guess mothers do these kinds of things to daughters.

Jessica also found that her cancer increased the strain in her relationship with her son. He was a senior in high school at the time and was struggling with a college decision.

I was a little upset about it because I didn't get a definite reaction from him, and we had always been pretty close. I didn't really know how to judge what he said and what he didn't say. I guess I was more upset about what he didn't say. You take a kid that's 18 years old and he's making a college decision, and he's got all of these things going on in his life, and his mother has breast cancer. How many do you know who are going to be comfortable talking about it? He was avoiding it more than anything. He didn't ignore me, but he didn't recognize my feelings, what I was thinking about, or what I was going through. I can remember telling my husband, "I don't understand why he is the way he is." But eventually, I found out that he really did care but just didn't know exactly how to handle it. He went out and bought me one of those beautiful cards—very emotional—that said all the things he didn't know how to say. That just took care of it more or less. We began to talk a little bit more and little by little it worked out.

I think part of it was that he was in the process of trying to separate himself from me and grow up, and he wanted me to let him do that. At the same time, I wanted him to still be close to me, because I felt like I needed him. That was a hard time for me, because when I was recuperating, he wasn't around.

In terms of the impact the cancer experience has had on her, Jessica says the following.

You know, there are two kinds of people when it comes to cancer: the people that keep themselves going and the other ones that sit down and complain because it happened to them, and nobody understands, and nobody cares. I didn't want to be like that. I don't want to wear a label. I mean, you never forget it. There's always something in the news that brings back certain feelings. It's always there, but you don't have to dwell on it. You don't have to let it control your life.

I just decided that I was going to try to focus on the better things. I didn't want to be negative. I have tried to appreciate my life a little more. I think I value my life and the people I'm close to more than I did before. I think it does make you stop and think about the positive—about what's important. Sometimes I lapse back into worrying about things that it's just not fruitful to worry about. But for the most part, I do value life.

Some people think that you have to accept it, and you have to fight it. I think I have a fight that's there. I wouldn't want to go through it if it happens again, but I guess I know if I had to, I would do everything I could. Some people give me the impression that they fight it every day. I don't know that I do. I don't have that attitude that I have to fight cancer the rest of my life. I feel like it's gone.

CASE 2: BETH

Beth, like many women of her generation, devoted her life to her home and family. She had five children, and she and her husband were very busy through the course of their marriage meeting the needs of their children. In fact, the children had been the focus of their marriage. Even on their 25th wedding anniversary, when they went away for a weekend, they both worried about the kids the whole time! At age 51, Beth had been married for 30 years, and her children were starting to leave home. Her youngest child was still in high school, and her oldest was married. Beth's parents were both deceased.

One day, Beth rolled over in bed, and felt something "a little different." She decided that it felt like a muscle, and decided not to pay any attention to it. When it didn't go away, however, she asked her husband what he thought.

> He said, "That's a lump, Beth!" But I thought, "he's overreacting." So then I asked my two daughters, and they definitely thought it was different. So I went to the doctor.

Beth's doctor said he didn't think it was anything, but sent her to a surgeon, "just as a precaution."

> He examined me, and then he sat down. And I thought, "I'm in deep trouble." When a doctor sits down and says, "Now, Dear . . .," you know you're in trouble.

The surgeon explained the one-step procedure to her. "I'm going to take you in, and remove the lump and examine the lump right there. If it's malignant, I take the breast off, right there." He advised against lumpectomy. He told her that she could go to another doctor and get a second opinion, but Beth said, "Well, I'll have to go with your opinion. If it's malignant, take it, because with a lumpectomy, you're living with a time bomb." Beth went into the hospital for her biopsy the very next day, only 2 days following her initial visit with her gynecologist.

> I was lying there thinking, "Well, if I'm going to die, whatever happens, I'm going to live for at least 2 more years, until Mary gets into college, because she needs me." I had to be there for Mary. Also, my husband looked scared to death. So I thought, "Well, I have to be strong for him." And now my oldest daughter, she was a wreck. I thought, "I have to stay calm. I can't show any signs that I'm a wreck too!" Just the look on their faces made me think, "My God! I can't go anywhere!"

Beth felt the need to curb her own reactions to her surgery to be strong for her husband and daughters. The next day, Beth had a modified radical mastectomy.

> I remember waking up and realizing that the breast was gone, and I was feeling kind of down in the dumps. My oldest daughter came in and said, "Mom, look at it this way, you could have lost your teeth!" This was a joke between us because as I started to get older, my mouth dropped, and when I smiled, I showed every tooth in my mouth. So I used to say, "Take care of your teeth, because when you get older, you show them all." So when she said, "You could have lost your teeth," that cracked me up. So that helped.

When Beth came home from the hospital, she experienced both anger and sadness.

> I can remember standing in the shower one day and thinking, "This really stinks!" And "Why me, God? I'm a good person. I go to church every Sunday." My reaction was, a part of my body is gone. And it was devastating! I mean I'm not a vain person or one that thought their body was great or anything like that. But it's a part of your body that's gone that was there for so long, and all of a sudden, it's not there. And you feel devastated. It's part of your femininity.

She also felt a strong sense of hope, however,

> I never really thought about it afterward. It's strange. Call it premonitions or whatever, but in my own mind, from right after the operation, I knew I was going to be all right. Whether it was that someone told me, whether it was God, I don't know. I just felt, I'm going to be fine.

Beth used her strong faith to help her make some meaning of her experience with breast cancer. "I thought, God did this for a reason. He meant me to do something good for other people. He wants me to go out and talk to people and to help other people." So Beth became a volunteer in the American Cancer Society's Reach to Recovery program.

Beth feels that her marriage is stronger as a result of her breast cancer.

> My life was so busy before, I honestly didn't have time to think about things. I was too busy trying to do the wash, clean the house, and just keep up with the activities of the family. Now, I have a totally different attitude about my husband. I appreciate him more. He was a big help to me when I needed him. And I realized how much he loved me. Which is good, when you're 51, to realize that he still loves you. He thought, "I could have lost Beth." And he appreciates me more. Before that, we were too busy to tell each other these things. We took each other for granted. But after the operation, I realized that all he cared about was that I was alive.

Although Beth's husband was not bothered by her postsurgical appearance, Beth was.

> It was me more than him. He didn't care. I would hide myself and so on, and he would say, "Beth, you're being silly!" It didn't bother him. Then, I began to gradually forget about it. But it took years. Two or 3 years.

About 2 years after her operation, Beth decided to have reconstruction.

> All I did was complain. I couldn't wear anything with a V-neck, because I had this hole. If I wore a scoop neck, I couldn't bend over. I couldn't find a bathing suit. I couldn't wear any sundresses. My daughter encouraged me to have the implant. She knew somebody who had had one and was really happy with it, and she pushed me into it. Now I'm happier in my clothes. There's no problem. I can wear what I want to wear. My plastic surgeon encouraged me to come back to have the other breast lifted, and I was scheduled to go in for that, but my husband didn't want me to. "Beth" he said, "Leave it alone! If anything happens . . . Leave it alone!" So I said, "Fine."

Beth's youngest daughter was thinking about going into nursing and took a very clinical attitude to her mother's illness. "She was very interested in it at the time. She wrote a paper on breast cancer in one of her courses in high school. She also did one in college."

Beth's attitude toward women has changed since her own experience with breast cancer and her volunteer work with Reach to Recovery. Before her experience with breast cancer, Beth was more "annoyed" by women who were "pushy."

> They would get on my nerves, because they were always pushing their kids. But, then, after visiting all these different women, I thought, "Women are great! They are strong. They are really good."

As a result of coping with breast cancer, Beth has come to appreciate her own personal strength and that of other women who have coped with this disease.

CASE 3: SANDRA

Sandra was a suburban homemaker, married to a very successful business-man, when she first noticed a lump in her breast. At the time, Sandra was 40 and had four children, ranging in age from 10 to 20 years. Like many women in the postwar years, Sandra had thought that she would be satisfied with a life devoted to husband and children. She found herself increasingly dissatisfied, however, and decided to pursue a career when her children were old enough to manage without her. Shortly before her 40th birthday, she had enrolled in a program that would prepare her to become a teacher.

Sandra came from a large but not very close family. This family had some serious dysfunctions that later affected Sandra's ability to cope with her breast cancer. Like many children of families with problems, Sandra became the "successful" child, representing her family to the outside world in a positive way. This was accompanied by a stifling of her true feelings and a pattern of poor communication with others. When she married, she repeated this pattern, and never developed a good pattern of communication with her husband or children. Instead, she focused on presenting a "good" picture of how things were.

When Sandra first discovered a lump in her breast, she wasn't terribly concerned.

> I found a lump in my breast, and saw my gynecologist about it. He decided that it wasn't anything to be concerned about. Then, I noticed that it had changed. It began to grow in size, and it began to bother me. So I went and had a needle biopsy done. I didn't discuss it with my husband. I didn't feel it was important to worry him about it until we had something to worry about. I waited for the call, and the doctor called one night when I was putting the children to bed, which is a terrible time to call anybody. You know, the magnitude of the whole thing did not really come in on me then. I just wanted to digest it. The next day, I took my husband and went to see the doctor. He talked about what we could do. He really was quite helpful. We talked about mastectomy and breast reconstruction. He said, "Well, no one has really had reconstruction." I found this to be rather shortsighted. So I called a surgeon I knew of, and he mapped out a plan for me. "We'll do an incisional biopsy and a bone scan, and we'll wait for the diagnosis, then I'll do the surgery, and then you'll come back in the future, and we'll do breast reconstruction." I felt much more at ease in his care, and so I decided to switch and go to this physician. And it certainly was a very good choice.

mom is ~~most~~ emotionally unavailable
at time when certainty is
highest

118   *Breast Cancer in the Life Course*

Two weeks later, Sandra had a mastectomy.

> I was in school at the time, and I had to take a final exam. I had to go to the instructor and explain what the situation was, and it was very difficult for me to say it. I mean, just in saying it, there was a reality in it. I did take the exam, and it was probably good because it gave me something to concentrate on.

Sandra believes that women need an advocate to help them cope with this experience.

> You really do need a mentor at that time. You're all caught up in the moment, and it's so difficult to make any kind of decision. You need an advocate to help you sort out all this information that you get, and someone to put their arms around you and give you a good hug. You need time. Time to sort it out, to prepare yourself for the future, and to come to terms with it.

Sandra feels that she could have benefited from some outside support to handle her feelings about the cancer and its treatment.

> I think I probably kept a lot of feelings inside. I didn't want to frighten my husband or my family, and I didn't want to frighten myself. It wasn't that I didn't accept it and go on with my life. But I didn't talk about it a lot. We probably should have sought some sort of professional help. Not that I was having a great deal of difficulty with coping, but it would have been better for me to speak with an objective individual instead of having to burden anyone in my family or a friend. I think the enormity of having cancer, I don't care what kind it is, is such that for people to make the adjustments, professional help would be good. It would help you feel that you are getting better, and there are people there helping you to do that.

Seven positive lymph nodes were found at Sandra's surgery, and a course of chemotherapy was recommended. This proved very difficult for Sandra.

> I was strong. I jogged and was very physically active. But chemotherapy really did zap my energy enormously. I lost all my hair, which, in the beginning, for about a week, was a problem. I bought a wig. But that was the least of my problems. The chemotherapy is a hormonal manipulator. And I went through a premature menopause. I really didn't understand what was happening to me. I didn't get proper information about hot flashes. I was up every night, and I was exhausted. I think quite frankly that the hormonal manipulation took more of a toll than the mastectomy did. Because you do lose your femininity. You really are like a 75-year-old woman. Your libido is squished. You have vaginal dryness.

Sandra and her husband were unable to communicate about her reaction to chemotherapy.

> My husband and I never discussed this. It's really difficult for him whenever I bring it up. I think he was frightened. I'm only able to assume this, because I have no way of knowing. There was nothing that he could deal with. If he

could call the doctor, or if he could take me out to dinner, that would be fine. He would never go to chemotherapy with me, but he would call me and say, "How are you today?" and I would usually say, "I'm OK." We were protecting each other. That's not unusual in our relationship. If it is something emotional, it's just real difficult for us to sit down and talk about it.

Sandra was able to discuss her illness with her children, however.

It was important for me to discuss it with them. I told them that I was going to the hospital, and what I was going to have done, and that I was going to be okay. And periodically, since then, I say to them, "Oh, I just had a doctor's checkup and everything is great." I'm not sure they wanted to sit down and talk about it. But I gave them the information, and if they wanted to go further, they could choose to do that. I talked to my daughter about having a mammogram and doing self exams. I think she worries more than the others. My older son was having his own problems at that time, and he was so wrapped up in himself I really don't think he thought about it. I never covered myself up. They would see it, and we would talk about it. I tried to be as matter of fact as I could. I would reassure them. I think it's very important to be straightforward with kids, because kids know when something isn't right. They know when there is all that whispering on the telephone, and people hiding in closets and crying. I didn't want them to worry about it.

I tried very hard not to need anything special. Which is probably not a good thing, in retrospect. There's no question that you should reach out and ask, "Please help me. I don't feel well today. Give me a little special attention." But that didn't happen.

Sandra did receive support from her brothers and sisters, and some of her friends.

My brothers and sisters all called me, and my friends were very supportive. I had one friend who had had a mastectomy years before, but she had never discussed it with me. I began to talk about it and ask her questions, and she opened up and was very supportive to me. Of all the people that I came in contact with, there was only one woman who I realized was so uncomfortable with this that she chose to stay away. It was almost as though I had a contagious disease. She brought a cake one day, but I could tell she really didn't want to spend any time with me. I just chose in the future not to pursue that relationship. I have another friend who is older than I am. We're very close, but in her world, you just don't discuss things like breast cancer in public. I tried to talk to her about it, but she found that kind of a brash thing. She finds it too personal—very difficult to share.

About a year after her surgery, Sandra had a second mastectomy for preventative reasons and then had breast reconstruction. Because of her style of coping and her lack of intimate family support, Sandra had bottled up her feelings for more than a year when she completed her second surgery. At that point, she describes herself as "one angry lady."

I was trying to keep a lid on everything and do what I was supposed to do and not worry anybody. I think a lot of it was that I kept putting off dealing with it. We can only deal with one thing at a time. I did go through a terrific problem when it finally all kind of came crashing in on me. Years, not months. Years. I remember sitting on the patio outside after I came home from the breast reconstruction, and I realized that I'd spent my entire life trying to do things for others, especially my family, to gain their love. My existence was making everybody happy. And the revelation was that it wasn't getting me anywhere. That was a very down time. That was the bottom when I came to that realization. Believe me, if I had a gun, I would have blown my brains out. I was really low.

But, see, I didn't have the gun, so I had to go on living. And, if I was going to go on living, I was going to make the best of it. I was going to be a participant rather than let it happen to me. I decided that if that was the way it was going to be, there were certain things—expectations—that I could see just weren't going to happen. And if I was going to continue to seek what wasn't going to happen, I was going to be unhappy. You know, as you get older, if you hang onto the things that you want when you're 20, you're going to be sorely disappointed. There are certain doors that shut. Whether it be the fact that you can't go back to medical school at the age of 60, or that the child that wasn't nurtured properly isn't going to be whatever you wanted him to be. These things aren't going to happen. You have to let go of some of that. So I learned to go with what I have and get on with it.

Sandra emerged from her difficult experience with cancer and its treatment with some new personal strengths and goals.

I came out of the other end a different person. I didn't have the anger anymore. I let go of the upset and the rage that maybe I took into this illness with me. Now it didn't happen right away. It's just been a steady climb up.

Sandra indicates that she is as comfortable now with her body as she was before her surgeries.

I don't think I've ever been very comfortable with my body. My brothers and sisters used to tease me all the time when I was little about being fat. They called me names. So I guess I've never been terribly happy with my body. The fact that I lost the breasts, when I would go to the gym or to a dressing room, I would be uncomfortable about that in the beginning. But now I can go and feel that I don't stand out in the crowd. I'm not concerned now that if somebody does see me that it's going to freak me out or that it's going to freak them out either. I mean, I would be able to answer their questions.

She has not accepted the loss of sexuality, however, which resulted from the chemotherapy.

As far as my husband is concerned, we really have no sexual relationship, and that's really sad. I don't have those hormones there, and that's tough. I've been to a couple of gynecologists and asked them this question. I think I am looking for someone to say "yes" to estrogen replacement therapy. Actually, I am looking for someone to sit down and talk to me about it. To consider my concerns and to say, "Yes, they are real." To say, "Look, this is a problem. I know what you're going through. I know it's not easy." Something. Something! Because even the oncologists have a difficult time talking about this. They just sort of shake their heads.

Her experience with breast cancer has brought Sandra in touch with the issue of mortality.

With breast cancer, you certainly come in touch with your mortality. I know that I had experiences, just awful experiences, where I had come in touch with mortality. That I was not going to live forever. The fact is that somebody says, "Hey, this is something that may shorten your life." You have to let go of so much garbage in your life! I mean there just isn't time for it! Somebody has touched you and said, "Hey, listen up! Don't be petty. Don't waste time on details that just don't make any difference at all!." I mean, most of it's been just so much time mucked down in nonsense. You just have to learn to forget about it. It's not worth the time.

As a result of this realization, Sandra has been searching for a way she can make a more meaningful contribution. She serves as a Reach to Recovery volunteer and would like to take up a teaching job.

So it's, "What do I want to do with the next 20 years?" I want to do something else. I'm not very happy just filling my hours. I have to make a commitment. Now I have my children raised. But then my husband says, "No, if you get a full-time job, then we can't travel." You know, men and women reach different stages at different times. He's ready to stop doing everything and go to Arizona to play tennis. And I have all the time and energy to devote to these things I want to do. So, there's a little conflict there, and we have to figure out how to resolve it.

Looking back on her experience with breast cancer, Sandra feels that there have been many positives which have come out for her.

I do feel that I'm a much stronger person. From the experience I've gone through, I know that I can get through most anything. I guess from the beginning, I was really a survivor. I trust myself and my coping. And I enjoy the physical aspects of life more now. Things that I never did take time for before, like taking an hour and going for a walk. These are important things. Now, it's OK if I want to go and get a facial. Taking care of myself. And I do laugh a lot. I can be very silly! And that's important too.

THEMES OF MIDLIFE WOMEN WITH BREAST CANCER: PART ONE

Jessica, Beth, and Sandra provide examples of midlife women with breast cancer struggling with the issues of body image, marriage, and relationships with adolescent children. In this section, these themes are discussed as they interact with the breast cancer tasks of maintaining a satisfactory body image and sexual relationships, managing psychological reactions such as anger and depression, and adapting to role shifts. Additional quotations from Sarah (age 42), Lynn (age 42), Joan (age 48), Ethel (age 52), Sylvia (age 52), and Marian (age 56) are used to illustrate these issues more fully.

Body Image

Although body image was an issue for most of the women in our study who had mastectomies, it was especially salient for the midlife women. Even without the possible disfigurement of breast cancer surgery, women at this life stage are experiencing physical changes associated with aging. The task of preserving a satisfactory body image for postmastectomy patients interacts with the women's life stage task of adapting to an aging body.

Body image has been described as a "mental picture of one's own body—the way in which the body appears to the self. It implies "a personal investment in various parts of the body" (Woods, 1979, p. 324). Both men and women experience changes in body image in midlife. Neugarten (1975), who interviewed 100 men and women, aged 45 to 55, found an increased sense of physical vulnerability, resulting in a form of "body monitoring," in which the middle-aged adult develops protective strategies to maintain the body. This issue of body image emerged as "typical of middle adulthood," and appeared in different ways, if at all, in younger or older adults (Colarusso & Nemiroff, 1981, p. 50).

In American society there is even less social acceptability of the physical aging process in women than in men. Meyerowitz, et al. (1988) report that middle-aged women are already labeled as less attractive and physically unappealing. "Although middle aged men may still be seen as attractive and sexual, prevailing sociocultural views equate female sexual desirability with a youthful body" (Colarusso & Nemiroff, 1981, p. 142). Consequently, women appear to have a more prolonged preoccupation with the loss of youth and the physical signs of aging. The middle-aged woman is increasingly aware of changes in her appearance and energy level—her relationship with her body is changing. Graying hair, weight gain, greater difficulty in recuperating from physical exertion, and menopause are some of the physiological indices of aging (Notman, 1980).

In addition to this normal aging process, mastectomy patients have to adapt to surgical removal of a body part that is closely associated with sexuality and attractiveness in our culture. When there is a discrepancy between the way in which a woman has mentally pictured her body and the way in which she currently perceives it, anxiety can be aroused. A distortion of her customary body image can be viewed as a distortion of self. The sudden onset of a serious illness like breast cancer can induce "feelings of loss of control over one's physical well-being and of betrayal by one's body" (Euster, 1979, p. 252).

Because for many women the breast represents a basic source of feminine identification, physical wholeness, and attractiveness, "the loss of the breast has the potential for shattering a woman's body image" (Euster, 1979, p. 253). Because of this change in body image, many women feel they have lost a part of themselves and experience uncertainty about their identity. Three years postmastectomy, Jessica is still adjusting to an altered body image that has slowed her down and made her less interested in physical activity. Before breast cancer, Jessica identified herself as a physically active person. Beth says, "A part of my body was gone. It was devastating!" Beth also emphasizes the sexual meaning of the breast ("It's part of your femininity"). One single woman we interviewed (see case study on Wanda in chapter 5) could not look at herself for 3 years and when she did, she felt "it was shocking and sad." Another single woman (see case study on Gwen in chapter 5) is equally unhappy with her body image since her mastectomy ("It's so ugly!").

Kushner (1975) found that postmenopausal married women, whose youth and sexual attractiveness have begun to fade, were more upset by the loss of a breast than young married women. For example, Marian (age 56), diagnosed with breast cancer at age 56, worried about her body image following her mastectomy.

> When I see attractive women on television in skimpy things with beautiful bosoms, I think, "Geez, did I used to look like that?" Because when it's there it's natural, and you don't give that much thought to it. All of a sudden you don't have it [breast] and then you worry. "What did I look like? Am I ever going to look normal again?" I was super careful about how every little thing looked—was this too low, was this too high? I was very intimidated about every which way I looked and every which way I moved.

Physiological signs of aging are experienced as narcissistic injury by both men and women, but "Women experience the physical effects of the aspects of aging primarily as a threat to their attractiveness to men" (Mann, 1980, p. 131). This focus on attractiveness to partners applies as well to the postmastectomy patient, who may fear rejection because of bodily distortion. In one breast cancer study, "some women projected their own feelings of unacceptability to men whom they felt judged women on the basis of their breasts" (Woods, 1979, p. 325).

Beth hid her mastectomy scar from her husband for several years, even though he was not bothered by it. In fact, it was her husband who discouraged her from having her remaining breast "lifted" following reconstruction. Jessica also was "a little bit uncomfortable" having her husband see her the first time. In Marian's case, she asked her husband how he felt about reconstruction. He asked, "Are you going to do it for me?" Marian said, "I would do it because I would hope it would please you." Her husband replied, "Well, don't do it for me. We've been married for 35 years. I'm not concerned. You are who you are with or without a breast." Despite these reassurances, Marian had breast reconstruction.

Perhaps Marian and Beth were also concerned with the effect of the loss of a breast on their self-esteem, as women are socialized in our culture to value highly their physical appearance. How women appear to one another may also gain them status in the world of other women. Jessica says of reconstruction, "It makes you feel a whole lot better about yourself." Jessica has experienced a changed body image ("I have an ugly keloid scar. . . . I have put on some weight"), but she seems more concerned with how she looks to others. ("I'm my own worst critic, and I can stand there and look this way and that, and I don't think anybody could tell").

In Sandra's case, she did not feel very good about her body before her mastectomy ("I don't think I've ever been very comfortable about my body"). As a result, she seemed to have fewer problems adjusting to a changed body image after mastectomy. In fact, she may be more comfortable now than before her surgery.

Another midlife woman who had a mastectomy found that coping with the loss of a breast and, consequently, a refocus on body image in midlife helped her to feel more positive about her body. She appreciates her body more since her bilateral mastectomies than she ever did before.

> I think everybody just takes [her] body for granted. Up until that point you just accept everything you've got—all your parts. And once you have a mastectomy, then you realize. . . . I want to look the best I can with what I have. I do feel that I have better posture because now I'm aware that I don't have anything here and I want to make sure that I look right. Before I thought "What difference does it make if I wear sloppy clothes—who wants to look at me anyhow?" Now I kind of feel differently. . . . I just know now I'm happy with myself. I'm happy with the way I look. Maybe I wasn't before—I don't know. But I know that when I put something on I'm going to look good in it.
>
> Ethel, age 52

For the midlife woman, an experience with breast cancer can interact with concern about physical aging in two different ways. Some women like Beth, Jessica, and Marian struggle to maintain a positive body image following a mastectomy. Other women, like Sandra and Ethel, have used the opportunity to refocus on body issues and to become more interested, comfortable, and relaxed with their bodies. Reconstructing a new physical sense of themselves is an extremely important area for midlife women, regardless of their life-style or level of sexual involvement. Whether single or married, today's midlife women are part of a cohort that was heavily influenced by physical appearance as a basis for their self-image and self-esteem. For the midlife woman coping with breast cancer, the struggles in adapting to an altered body image should not be underestimated.

Marriage

Research on the family life cycle (Carter & McGoldrick, 1980) indicates that one of the developmental tasks confronting the midlife couple is renegotiation of their marital roles. Because children are growing up and, in some cases, leaving the home, the couple must begin to refocus their energies away from their role as parents and decide how they want to spend their time. If one partner wants to spend more time together and the other wants more private time, frustration, anger and depression can result. When the stresses inherent in a disease such as breast cancer are superimposed on a marriage already undergoing major changes, the tension can become extreme. From "the time of initial diagnosis, through treatment and adjustment, when a woman is grieving her loss and when her mate is also grieving that loss, the cancer crisis does strain their relationship, sometimes to the breaking point" (Johnson, 1987, p. 110).

In Sandra's case, communication problems were a major stumbling block in negotiating new marital roles at midlife as well as in integrating the couple's reaction to the breast cancer experience. Other midlife women also experienced communication problems, with wives describing their husbands' inability to help. The following examples describe these difficulties.

> My husband was more frightened by my emotional changes than the physical change in my body. Anything that is mental or emotional is hard for him— because he can't fix it. Men don't want to feel helpless. Soon after my mastectomy he took a book out from the library on the emotional changes of cancer patients, but we didn't discuss emotional issues between us. I don't think it's [the marriage] going to get any better. That's a shame. I've tried to get him to go for therapy. . . . I just really feel if we could just open up those lines of communication that it might make it better . . . from wherever he comes, whatever world he comes from that's just not what he's comfortable with.

> Lynn, age 42

> You know, his [the husband's] problem is worrying about me and not being able to do anything. And this is typical of all men, I believe. They don't . . .

their wives are suffering with something . . . what can they do? They can't do anything. And he would say to me, "What can I do for you? . . . What can I do? . . . How can I help?" And so many times I was tempted to say, "Just leave me alone. Just don't make me think. . . . Don't make me talk. . . . Just leave me alone." But I couldn't do that to him.

Marian, age 56

[My husband] could never express his true feelings as far as being worried. I knew that he was very upset [about the breast cancer]. But he would never talk about it. He could never express his feelings. . . . I knew he was upset when he would snap at me. I would talk to him and say, "You know I'm going to live forever." He would say "Well, of course you are." But I could tell by his tone of voice that he really didn't think I was going to be all right. Cancer scared him . . . but he was trying to assure me that I was OK.

Ethel, age 52

I can't share with my husband; he just doesn't know how. He's a good person, but he just does not know how. It's not his—I don't want to burden him. I don't want to be "the menopausal mother" that's got all these crazy thoughts going on in her mind. . . . I cry, and I hope. . . . [I] don't look to my husband—[I] don't tell him to do anything. [I] don't tell him anything.

Sylvia, age 52

These quotations suggest that men may think that sharing their feelings makes them vulnerable in a relationship (Gilligan, 1982b; Johnson, 1987; Miller, 1986). These breast cancer patients wanted to share their feelings with their husbands and receive emotional support. Their husbands were eager to provide concrete support and verbal reassurance but were not responsive enough to their wives' emotional needs. Smith et al. (1985) report that the most beneficial support activity for women with breast cancer was socioemotional (listening to or talking with their wives about the disease), whereas supportive task activities were regarded as less important.

Nor does it seem that these women were able to be direct in expressing what they needed ("I don't want to burden him"). In a traditional marriage, husbands are responsible for the instrumental tasks (e.g., earning a living), whereas wives are responsible for the socioemotional tasks (Parsons, 1949) Problems arise in this type of marriage when the wife needs socioemotional support. The husband may be incapable of providing this type of support. In the marriages described earlier, the husband responded in a traditional way—doing things—but was at a loss in how to provide emotional support. Wives used to providing emotional support were not sure how to ask for it. Perhaps women also tend to withdraw because of their increased anxiety over their changing body image and their fear that their husbands cannot bear to look at them. (Asken, 1975; Witkin, 1979). Breast cancer patients may be less likely than they normally might be to share their concerns with their spouse. A husband may also be afraid of hurting his wife emotionally by saying or doing the "wrong thing" or of accidentally hurting her physically, especially during love making (Johnson, 1987). Asken (1975) and Witkin (1979) discuss implications of the "mastectomy bind" for both the patient and her husband. The husband of a breast cancer patient may withdraw emotionally because he is unsure of how to respond, partly out of guilt because he may feel he failed to help his wife. Each partner needs physical and emotional caring from the other, but finds it too risky to express these needs. Midlife is a difficult time for marriages, which are naturally undergoing role shifts. Breast cancer at this time adds a new set of strains on a couple that can further estrange the partners, particularly when the wife has been the provider of socioemotional support.

Initiating or maintaining open communication seems to be critical for couples in coping successfully with a crisis such as breast cancer. According to Seltzer (1988), the sexual difficulties that some couples face following mastectomy are the result of each spouse being cautious and uncertain about the needs and feelings of the other. Couples are often afraid to discuss feelings openly because they worry about making each other more upset. Furthermore, couples coping with a cancer experience tend to "show protectiveness toward their mates" (Leiber, Plumb, Gestenzang, & Holland, 1976, p. 386; Naysmith, Hinton, Meridith, Mackes, & Berry, 1983).

A diagnosis of breast cancer, however, actually strengthened the marital unit in some cases by enabling the couple to feel more precious to each other—facilitating intimacy between the partners. In Beth's view, her marital relationship has grown stronger since her diagnosis with breast cancer. Both she and her husband appreciate each other more. Since her mastectomy Beth believes that they have grown closer because they share a deeper realization of their love for one another. Before her surgery this couple took each other for granted, but afterward realized how precious they were to each other and began enjoying the increased time they had together as a couple. Another midlife woman describes the following sentiment.

> Now I can appreciate what happens to older couples who suffer heart attacks. . . . And these people become even more dear, because you realize how vulnerable they are. . . .

Jessica had strong support from her husband, including the "moral support" that she suspects most husbands do not provide. It is interesting to note that Jessica's marriage was fairly new, and was not going through a change of long-standing patterns at the same time.

Another midlife woman (Marian, 56), who found her marriage strengthened by the cancer experience, points out that at this stage of life, work is becoming less important to her husband.

> Work is no longer a driving force to him. He feels like he can say sometimes, "The hell with it! My wife comes first—There are more important things than the company."

Couples in midlife are at a different point (from those in early adulthood) in their lives regarding their careers. Many men are no longer "climbing the corporate structure but are more settled in a career or job (Levinson et al., 1978). Perhaps it is easier for these midlife husbands to put their work "on a back burner" during a medical crisis. Marian also found her husband more supportive of her desire to work outside the home after her experience with cancer. Further, Marian's experience seems to have helped her separate out "who she is" as she defines herself more by her own experience and less by her marital partner.

We found that married midlife women relied heavily on their husbands for a sense of being loved and esteemed (Holland & Mastrovito, 1980; Northouse, 1988). Beth's husband was not turned off by her appearance. Jessica's husband moved at a pace at which she was comfortable ("He didn't force me to face the fact of him looking at me . . . and that helped"). Perhaps the best example of this type of support came from another midlife womanwho had been married for 22 years at the time of her diagnosis.

> I'm very fortunate. I have a very supportive husband and he was there for me all the time. In fact, when I had to have chemotherapy after the second mastectomy, he went to every chemotherapy session with me, which I appreciated. I lost my hair after a while, and he said something that was really good. After I was bald and everything, he said, "You know, there's something very sexy about you being bald." And that really made me feel *so* good.

Nearly all of the married midlife women we interviewed discussed the effects of breast cancer on their marriage. Because the marital relationship may be more vulnerable at midlife, the tasks of coping with breast cancer (changing roles, dealing with feelings) interact with the task of renegotiating the marital contract. The previous role relationships within the marital dyad (regarding dependency needs) may determine what happens during the couple's experience with breast cancer. In cases in which the woman has "taken care" of her husband, the marital balance was upset so that neither partner could meet the other's needs. In some cases, a diagnosis with breast cancer served to make a poor marriage more difficult (e.g., Sandra and Sylvia).

In other cases, however, marriages were changed for the better. In Marian's case, when breast cancer upset the previously established marital balance, this couple was able to renegotiate their roles and move in a positive direction toward increased support and communication. In Beth's case the experience with cancer helped them renegotiate their marriage to become more couple focused and less child focused. Although Beth and her husband had a rewarding relationship before their experience with breast cancer, they grew closer, appreciated each other more, and spent more time alone together following her mastectomy. Like any other life crisis, breast cancer can be used positively to promote better adjustment. Reassessment of a relationship is often an outgrowth of life-threatening illness, bringing values into sharper focus (Holland & Mastrovito, 1980).

In a rewarding marriage partners feel that they can express their true feelings and needs, believing that their partner will attempt to meet those needs (Johnson, 1987). Jessica and her husband had discussed a way to be direct with one another to facilitate meeting each other's needs. In the case of Sandra, Ethel, and other women we interviewed, both partners seemed to have withdrawn from each other emotionally, creating a real block in marital communication. Partners may need to learn to be more direct with one another, and husbands may need to learn to respond to their wives' need for emotional support.

Relationships with Adolescent Children

The midlife woman with breast cancer is usually coping with adolescent children. Adolescent children may have an especially difficult time in coping with a mother's breast cancer because additional family responsibilities may be placed on them at a time when they are beginning to "emotionally withdraw from the family in order to establish their own identity" (Berger, 1984, p. 89; National Cancer Institute, 1984). Put another way, it has been said that cancer "creates an abrupt reversal of normal adolescent processes" because it "forces intensified contact with parents" at a time when the adolescent is "working on separation from family and establishing an individual identity" (Blumberg et al., 1982, p. 181). Although Baumann (1988) reports that most adolescents adapted successfully to their mother's experience with breast cancer, other research (National Cancer Foundation, 1977) indicates that adolescents who were aware of the diagnosis exhibited increased behavior problems.

Jessica expresses the conflict with dependence and independence experienced by adolescents and their parents when a crisis such as breast cancer is superimposed on adolescence. Her son's preparation for separation and "leaving the nest" conflicted with Jessica's special needs for closeness and support as she faced a life-threatening illness ("He was in the process of trying to separate himself from me and grow up . . . and I wanted him to still be close to me because I needed him").

Sandra didn't talk a lot about her cancer with her children but would reassure them that she was OK. By and large Sandra's children ignored her situation at the time of the diagnosis and mastectomy. Her teenaged son was "too much into himself to even think about it—he was dealing with his own problems in school." Sandra reported that her 14 year-old daughter

> did worry about me—she didn't say that then [at the time of diagnosis and mastectomy] but has said so since. She has told me, "I was really worried about you Mom. I worried about you from time to time."

Sandra's message to other women with breast cancer is that "Kids can't always let you know how they feel at the time because they're too frightened."

In Beth's case, her 16-year-old daughter was very concerned, but channeled her feelings and her concern into school projects on breast cancer, not into emotional support for Beth. This daughter is now a nurse, perhaps providing her patients the kind of support she could not provide her mother.

Another midlife woman reported that her relationship with her 18-year-old daughter (an only child) broke down after her surgery.

> I was very hurt by her. I was angry at her for not really being there for me—she should have been there with me. . . . But now, when I look back, the word cancer is so frightening—so frightening to young people.

It is important that midlife women who are coping with adolescent reactions to cancer understand that their teenagers will probably be unable to provide them with the emotional support that they may be wanting and expecting. (Jessica said her son "didn't recognize my feelings.") Although it seems important to tell the adolescent what is happening, it is also important not to expect this disclosure to help the teenager to have the "insights of an adult" or to offer support as another adult might do (Johnson, 1987).

Although our study is on women with breast cancer, and not on their children, we could not help noticing what seemed to be a high rate of problems in the teenaged daughters of our midlife interviewees. Joan was in her late 40s at the time of her diagnosis and had a 16-year-old daughter.

Joan reports how her mastectomy took place "in the time in her (daughter's) life [when] she was going to the prom. I guess she was a little bit resentful. Thirteen months after I had my mastectomy, I had a hysterectomy. This time, it was her junior prom, and she was getting a little annoyed with me." Following Joan's initial surgery, her teenaged daughter became quite ill with anorexia nervosa.

> My daughter was very, very ill, and at times I didn't know whether I was going to be able to handle that. She was anorexic . . . we went through a horrible period and at one point she was in and out of the hospital 25 weeks out of the year.

Sarah's daughter was 16 when Sarah had her second mastectomy. Sarah's daughter became anorexic in her first year of college and lost a lot of weight for about 1 year. "She [Sarah's daughter] said nothing was wrong, but I think it might have been a reaction [to the breast cancer]. Because she was really very concerned, and I really didn't know how to handle it."

In four cases (out of seven midlife interviewees who had adolescent daughters) an adolescent daughter had difficulty successfully negotiating the struggle of independence-dependence that is so crucial for developing a sense of identity. In two cases, within 1 year of their mother's diagnosis with breast cancer, the daughters developed anorexia nervosa. In the third case the daughter took up with an undesirable boyfriend, became pregnant, and dropped out of college. In a fourth case the 18-year-old daughter completely severed a relationship with her mother and moved in with her father because she was so frightened by the cancer.

When a disease like breast cancer strikes, anorexia nervosa can be a way of gaining control. A teenaged daughter's reaction to her mother's breast cancer experience could be an attempt to gain control over her own life when the family equilibrium has been upset, as well as a way to express concern and worry about her own body. A daughter might be extremely worried about her own sexual development, especially breast development, following her mother's breast cancer.

Because of fears in both adolescent girls and their mothers, it may be difficult for either the mother or her daughter to be open and supportive to one another. Because of her own physical aging, the midlife woman can be vulnerable to the sexual growth of her teenaged daughter. She may feel angry or jealous toward her daughter and be guilt ridden as a result. Concurrently, the daughter may experience guilt regarding her mother's illness because of her own budding sexuality. She may also experience anger toward her mother because she is aware of the possibility that she too may develop breast cancer (see case study on Nancy in chapter 3). Regardless of their reaction, this experience does not make it easy for mothers and daughters to share emotional reactions with one another.

Schain (1977) and Lichtman et al. (1984) found difficulties in the mother-daughter relationship following breast surgery. Because of their own fears about breast cancer, teenaged and adult daughters found it very stressful to relate to their mothers after breast cancer surgery (Schain, 1977).

From our interviews with midlife women who were mothers of adult children at the time of their diagnosis, it seemed that more often than not, adult sons and daughters provided physical and emotional support to their parent both during and after the crisis. Beth's adult children were extremely supportive of her throughout the process of her experience with breast cancer—from the diagnosis through her reconstruction. In fact it was her oldest daughter (age 23) who encouraged her to consider reconstructive surgery. For Beth having adult daughters was a godsend because she felt she could talk things over with them.

It may be easier for adult children who already have a more established sense of identity to support their parents during a crisis than it is for a teenager who is struggling to "break away" from home emotionally and establish a sense of self. Fischer (1986) found in her study of the mother-daughter relationship that most of the daughters said "the worst time in their relationships with their mothers was when they were teenagers," but as they matured and married with families of their own, their relationships with their mothers improved (Fischer, 1986, p. 45). Gould (1978) argues that midlife parents struggle to "keep that feeling of safety intact," which moves them toward "holding on to power" over their teenaged children. If adolescents are kept in the family, the parent can retain some of the feeling of safety that is slipping away with the death of parents and their own aging process (Gould, 1978, p. 225). This need to hold on to adolescents may be exacerbated by the woman's experience with breast cancer because she may want the family to grow closer and tighter as a result of her medical crisis. The adolescent child has to push harder to move toward independence, which creates added conflict and strain.

SUMMARY

Three themes have been explored in this part of the discussion on breast cancer in midlife women: body image, marriage, and relationships with adolescent children. Breast cancer treatment, and the resulting task of preserving a satisfactory body image, can interact with a midlife concern about physical aging in two different ways. Although most women (both single and married) felt they had to struggle to maintain a positive body image following mastectomy, a few women have used the increased opportunity to refocus on body issues to become more interested in, comfortable with, and relaxed with their bodies. Midlife women who have had mastectomies are struggling to reconstruct a new and positive physical sense of themselves, regardless of life style or level of sexual involvement. Because of the intersection of these two tasks, body image may be more important to midlife breast cancer patients than it is to women in other age groups.

Because the marital relationship may be more vulnerable at midlife, the tasks of coping with cancer, particularly managing psychological reactions and adapting to role shifts, interact with the midlife task of renegotiating the marital relationship. Some relationships that had a minimal amount of communication before the cancer experience become more difficult and troubled, whereas other relationships used the cancer experience as a catalyst to improve communication and increase the level of intimacy. Couples do best when they can be direct with each other in communicating their needs, and husbands are most helpful when they can respond to wives' need for emotional as well as task-oriented support.

Parents of adolescent children need to "let go" and help the children achieve autonomy. This task may be very difficult in light of a woman's need for increased support as she copes with the demands of breast cancer. Because of the breast cancer, families may be asking adolescent children to take on more responsibility or to intensify their contact with parents at a time when teens are trying to become independent. In our study, adolescent daughters had particular difficulty. It seems important that midlife women who are coping with adolescent's reactions to cancer understand that teenagers will probably be unable to provide their mothers with emotional support. Adult children in our sample were more likely to provide both physical and emotional support.

5 Experiencing Breast Cancer in Midlife: Part II

The case studies of Diane, Wanda, and Gwen provide further examples of how the breast cancer exerience affects women in midlife. Diane, age 46, and single was living a lesbian life-style and working as a high-level administrator when diagnosed with breast cancer. Diane had a modified radical mastectomy that determined that 80% of her lymph nodes had cancer involvement. She began a course of chemotherapy in the hospital that lasted 8 months, followed by a second type of chemotherapy, with concurrent radiation treatment. Diane supplemented conventional medical therapies with vitamins, imaging, massage, and healing therapy. Single, at age 47, Wanda was working as a travel agent when her breast cancer was discovered. Wanda's surgery was done in the mid-1970s when the common practice was to do a biopsy and if a carcinoma was found, to do a radical mastectomy immediately. Gwen, at age 59, was single and lived with an old friend at the time of her diagnosis. Gwen had been a teacher for many years but had gone into semiretirement from her profession just 1 month before her diagnosis. Gwen had a modified radical mastectomy followed by hormone-blocking treatment.

The voices of Diane, Wanda, and Gwen illustrate some important issues faced by many midlife women we interviwed. In midlife, adults face the fact that they have probably lived more years in the past than they will in the future. Diane, who was diagnosed with inflammatory breast cancer and given a little more than 2 years to live, decided to confront death by taking control of her own treatment. Gwen came to terms with her fear of dying when she thought she had a recurrence 1 year after the initial diagnosis, and, after working this through, no longer fears death.

Midlife is also thought to be a time of reassessment of one's life and a time of reprioritizing. Following her experience with breast cancer, Diane changed the way she was living in very fundamental ways by planning her social schedule before her work schedule. Gwen claims that her semiretirement coincided with midlife reassessment and her experience with breast cancer to help her learn to trust the ebb and flow of life—the process of living. At midlife, women tend to become more assertive and autonomous—they develop a new sense of self-reliance. Both Diane and Gwen are working harder at meeting their own needs.

Midlife adults search for opportunities in which they can feel appreciated and experience a personal sense of effectiveness—they want to achieve generativity. Gwen used her breast cancer experience to direct her energy toward developing workshops for women. Although at midlife women's relationships with mothers have often shifted into a pattern in which the mother has become more dependent on the midlife daughter for emotional or physical support, during Wanda's illness her mother took care of her. In contrast, Gwen did not count on her mother who was 93 years of age and lived at a distance, and Diane chose not to accept the support offered by her immediate family. In our study midlife women placed a heavy emphasis on friendships, although for a breast cancer patient this may mean taking a risk in terms of whether or not she will receive the support she wants and needs from her friends. For Diane, many of her friends were like family to her, although some friends were unable to deal with her life-threatening illness. Gwen received support from many friends following her mastectomy but also reported that some of her close friends "pulled back."

In the second section of this chapter, these themes of confronting death, reassessment of one's life, self-reliance, generativity, relationships with mothers, and friendships are explored as they intersect with the breast cancer tasks.

CASE 1: DIANE

Diane, a high-level administrator at age 46, had suffered a series of losses. An only child, she had been the primary caregiver for several elderly relatives. Within a year of the death of the last of these relatives, Diane had a diagnosis of breast cancer.

> I was exhausted! My work kept me traveling a lot. I would fly in to the airport and go straight to the nursing home. It was that kind of schedule. When the last one died, I was so tired I could barely get up in the morning. I mean, I'd just buried the third person, I'd just had pneumonia, but I knew there was something else going on. I was not afraid of cancer. I was completely convinced it was something wrong with my heart. I went to see the doctor for the first time in February. In May, I had a mammogram, and they read it as clean. So I said, "Well, that's not it." By September, I was so sick I couldn't even do a

2-mile hike! I had to lie down on the floor at work to rest! I mean, it was way beyond anything I'd ever experienced. I went back to the doctor's office and said, "The nipple's inverted. Something's wrong!" The doctor was not paying any attention. "Oh, don't worry about it. You had a mammogram in June. It was clean." I kept saying, "There's something wrong."

About a month later, I was at a conference with an old friend. She had had a double mastectomy the year before. I said, "You know, there's something wrong. I really don't feel good. I've been to the doctor. I've had a mammogram, but, the thing's inverted." And she screamed at me—literally stood up and screamed at me, "Get a second opinion! What are you doing? Get a second opinion!"

When she got back after her trip, Diane decided to have her doctor look at her breast one more time.

So I saw my doctor again as soon as I got back, and she turned white. It was the most scary thing I have ever lived through personally. She just went white and called the surgeon. The surgeon said, "I'm putting you in the hospital Monday morning." It was very frightening, because I was aware by then that I didn't have ordinary breast cancer. I had inflammatory breast cancer. I called my oldest and dearest friend and said, "I'm in big trouble!"

In 10 days, I went from being half convinced it was in my head—I just needed to get away from work and get a vacation—to realizing that I was likely to die. I saw several doctors, and all my friends were doing research, and they were saying things like, "You have a 2½-year life expectancy." The way they juggle time and statistics is very frightening!

Diane had a modified radical mastectomy, and it was found that 80% of her lymph nodes showed cancer involvement. She began a course of chemotherapy while still in the hospital. The first chemotherapy treatments lasted for 8 months.

So from then on, I was simply a sick person. The hair disappeared within about 10 days, and I would be violently sick every 3rd week, and then I would be OK again. We were doing treatments 2 out of 3 weeks, so I had 1 week in 3 where I'd be some semblance of a real person, and I could actually work!

This was followed by a second type of chemotherapy, with radiation treatment at the same time.

My doctor was very aggressive. He gave me the radiation while continuing chemotherapy, so that by the time that was over, I was incredibly sick. I still kept a modest work life going. Otherwise I would have gone crazy. My doctor wanted me to stay on the chemo for 18 months, but at the end of the first calendar year, I was so sick, I went in and said, "I'm done!" So I quit. I was convinced that my will to live was more important than the chemicals they were putting into me, and I was losing it. That was the hardest thing to do. I called a friend and said, "You've got to go with me, because I don't intend to be talked out of this." And when he saw the two of us in there, he said, "Well, your body is telling you something." So there was no argument about it.

Throughout her experience with cancer, Diane's main support came from her close friends. Like many lesbians, she has developed a network of women friends who has become like family to her.

> I have a lot of friends, and everyone called me on the phone and visited. Every weekend and on all the holidays, someone would come to visit. Some friends put together a standing order for flowers. Things like that mattered a great deal. So at some incredibly deep level I realized that I had family. I had incredibly close relations with several friends, and those relationships just got richer and richer. We have such a strong friendship network. One of my friends said, "This is going to be a group illness," and I think she was totally right. I was the first one of us to go down with something serious, and everybody had to think through what it meant. Psychologically, everybody learned a lot, and in their own ways, had to deal with things that are coming for them.

Diane did not seek support from her immediate family, although she did reach out to extended family. She also had a few friends who were not able to provide support at the time, although they were able to help her later.

> I had three old lovers who were incapable of relating at all. One just disappeared. One was supposed to visit and then canceled out. One just sent a couple of cards. We have since had several talks, but we haven't talked about the fact that she wasn't there for me. We've both chosen just to ignore that.

Diane had a hard time coping with the changes in her body.

> Oh God, suddenly you're totally disfigured! You're in pain, you look funny, and it hurts like hell. I put on 30 to 35 pounds. There was the sudden loss of the breast, about which I was ambivalent to start with. No hair. Your body is disintegrating! Your toenails come off. Your teeth chip off. Your bruises don't heal. Your skin looks like parchment. I went into menopause. My arm didn't function very well, because I had no nerve endings and no muscles. And it hurt for a long time, particularly after the radiation, because they burned it. So I not only had what was originally the stretching of the scars, but I had all the burns. I was convinced that I was totally unattractive. And I was. This is not my imagination. I'm not making this up. I looked like hell. Suddenly, I was middle-aged. My 40s, which I was expecting to be quite interesting, were gone.

She found the lesbian community to be accepting of her mastectomy, however,

> I went to a music festival. This is a completely lesbian kind of touch. Women there tend to wear clothes or not, as they feel like it. Lots of people are naked.

I'd known that when I got involved in that, I was going to have to make some decisions. Initially, I just wore a loose shirt. But by the second day, I said, "Oh, the hell with it!" and I went without a shirt at all. I did notice another woman there with a mastectomy and one with a double mastectomies. One of my friends said I looked "kinky", and she meant it as a compliment. My California friend just said, "Like everybody's into mutilation, so come on out!" So, there's a different context into which it gets fitted.

Diane coped with her very serious illness and poor prognosis by fighting back, not only with conventional medicine but with nonconventional therapies as well.

I took charge from day one. I had to heal. I decided that if you could grow a cancer, you could ungrow it. I was doing vitamins; I was doing exercise; I was doing imaging; I was doing a support group; I was doing laughing. You name it. Anything that made any sense to me, I was doing. I had a wonderful Indian healer who did a laying on of hands. I had massage therapy. I went to healing workshops and conferences. I've been a really active person in this other kind of healing. To me, that's been at least as important as the conventional medicine.

Diane has also been actively engaged in therapy to explore problems stemming from her childhood.

The most important thing is something I knew had to be done, which is that I had to deal with certain psychological material that was unfinished. The most arduous work I've done has been around childhood issues. That's just unrelenting and awful!

At the time of her interview, Diane had just turned 50. She is not in a long-term relationship, but she has gone back to dating. She feels that dating may be easier for a lesbian woman than for a heterosexual one, because "lesbian women are less addicted to fetishes in the body than men are."

Like so many cancer patients, Diane is frequently reminded of her disease.

I simply can't read an article, or see something on TV, or deal with my real life without triggering it. There is no way that I don't know that I'm still very much at risk, not only from the breast cancer but because the treatments I had left me at higher risk for other kinds of cancer. But I don't think you can handle it without going into denial.

Despite the knowledge of her risk, Diane cared for a close friend who eventually died from cancer.

I chose to make that journey with her. It was important. I know one of the things I legitimately have to give to people now is a kind of experience that a lot of people don't have.

When asked how her experience with cancer has changed her life, Diane responds as follows.

> I knew I had to start living in the present. Like a lot of high achievers, I lived way out ahead of myself. And I'm genuinely more positive about everything. I take more vacations. I don't feel guilty when I don't do something. I plan my social schedule first now and then my work schedule. That would never ever ever have happened if this had not happened. That's an enormous gain. I think cancer is an answer as well as a question. I don't recommend cancer to anybody, but it's like anything else. It's what you do with it that makes all the difference. It's a remarkable opportunity. There is enough in the literature and in the feminist community to make it a growth experience if you chose to use it that way.

CASE 2: WANDA

Single at age 47, Wanda decided to move out of the small town where she was raised, and to sample life in the "big city," Atlanta. She left behind her widowed mother, and lots of cousins, neices, and nephews. She also made a career shift from fashion consultant to work as a travel agent. She loved the stimulation of a big city, where she had the opportunity to "meet people from all over," and she loved her new job. She says, "I do love travel!"

Less than a year after the move, Wanda found a lump in her breast.

> I hadn't been there quite a year when I took a shower, and lay down on the bed, and I happened to put my hand on my breast and I felt something hard. So I called my doctor in my hometown, and he told me to come in the next day. At first, I didn't tell anybody. I blocked it out. Certainly I didn't tell my mother. My doctor examined me and scheduled me for a mammogram the next week. He called me in Atlanta and said I was going to be operated on. The next thing I remember, there was an empty bottle of wine on the kitchen counter!
>
> My doctor got me through very quickly. Too quickly for me, as it turned out, because he felt that women fall apart if they have too much time to think about it. As a result, I didn't get to meet the surgeon until the night before the surgery. Actually, I wouldn't have picked this surgeon. I never really had a chance to bond with him.

Wanda's surgery was done in the mid-1970s, when the common practice was to do biopsy, and if a carcinoma was found, to do a radical mastectomy immediately.

> When he [the surgeon] came in the night before the operation, he said to me, "Tell me something about yourself." And I didn't really tell him about myself. I should have said, "I'm 48, I'm single, and I live in Atlanta." I didn't do any of

that. I just told him how I found the lump. If I had told him that I was single, maybe he wouldn't have taken the muscles out. So I was angry at myself for not being assertive. I wasn't angry at the doctors. All the anger was on myself.

When the surgeon felt the lump, he said, "It's nothing." But I didn't say to myself, "Whoopee! It's nothing!" I knew it wasn't. You know, you have an instinct. After the surgery, I woke up and felt my bandage. Until then, I wasn't sure, but when you feel your bandage, you know. Mine went down to my waist!

Following her surgery, Wanda went to stay with her mother for several weeks. Her recovery was rapid. She was not depressed, and had no subsequent troubles with her arm. She attributes this to the exercises she began at the hospital and continued rigorously at home. She also feels the care her mother provided helped her heal quickly.

Although she [the mother] had cried some when I was in the hospital, when I got home, she didn't feel depressed. She was just very nurturing. She was glad to take care of me. And she was sunny enough. I stayed with her for 6 weeks, and she was just happy to have me there and be able to take care of me. It was never depressing around her, because she was just so happy to have a child to take care of again. A 48-year-old child! But she just enjoyed nurturing.

In describing her feelings about being nurtured at the age of 48, Wanda said the following.

Well, I needed her. I'll tell you what I needed her for—I didn't have an appetite and she said, "You're going to eat!" And she just had these marvelous dinners for me every night. Had I been alone, I would have been eating cottage cheese or tuna. The neighbors came and said, "You look marvelous! Your mother's taking good care of you!" So having my mother to feed me for 6 weeks, I'm sure I had a sparkle in my eye.

Wanda, however, was not able to express negative emotions while at her mother's house.

I read articles that say you're going to cry afterward. It didn't happen while I was with my mother 'cause I had someone around me. But when I went back to my apartment in Atlanta, I sat on the edge of my bed, and I cried. But it wasn't depression. It was, I guess, a letting out of everything.

Nor did she have a easy time developing a satisfactory body image.

It took me a few years to look at myself. I was afraid to look, and I remember asking a friend, "How am I going to look?" and she said, "You don't have to look." Even at the doctors, I sat with my eyes closed during the examinations. And you know, you don't need to look when you're dressing. You don't even have to look when you're bathing!

> When I did finally look, it was shocking and sad. When I saw how thin the skin was, and how it goes in with the muscles—I'll tell you, it was a good thing I waited 3 years!
>
> At my post-op checkup in the surgeon's office, he said, "See, I left it straight across here" [gesturing along the collar bone]. He was an older man, and he said, "See, I left it here, here, and here, so you can still wear a sundress!" That's what he said. I wonder how he thinks sundresses are made? I knew I could never wear those little slip sundresses again. And I felt a little sad about that. To this day, when I walk past a lingerie department, and I see these pretty little gowns, there is just a little sadness that I can't wear that. There's just pretty little summer things that I'll never be able to wear.

Wanda returned to her job in the travel office, and faced no discrimination because of her cancer.

> I was very fortunate. No one treated me any differently. I didn't see a look in anybody's eyes, like "Oh, poor Wanda!" I wasn't treated gingerly. Like I was wondering if I was going to get a look in people's eyes. I'm pretty perceptive. I can see if anybody is looking at me with a funny look. Nothing! I was really fortunate.

Although Wanda continued to date and to be active socially, she worried about how her illness and her operation would affect her relationships with men.

> The only thing any single woman thinks about is how she will be accepted by a male. At first, I was worried about how to tell men. But I read an article that said, "You don't have to tell anybody. It's nobody's business." And I took that approach. But later, I wanted to get a man's reaction. So I told two men, but I wasn't being that brave because I picked two men who I wasn't particularly interested in. It didn't matter to them. They both called me back. But it wasn't a true test, because I had nothing to lose. I knew they weren't my type.

Although this "test" was positive, Wanda still worries about rejection if she were to find a man who she is seriously interested her.

> If you really cared, you'd worry that that's going to be it. The moment of truth is how much you care for him, and how much the loss would be to you if he does turn away. The whole thing is if you stand to get hurt. If I get to the third date and I start to like him, then I know I'll have to tell him, and the fear will come in. I wouldn't have trouble telling, but it's how am I going to handle the hurt and the pain if something that looked promising all of a sudden gets cut off by that?

Perhaps because of this fear, Wanda has not had a relationship that has gotten past the crucial "third date" since mastectomy. Although she still hopes to get married some day, she realizes that, "At this age, I may very well never get married."

I have a good image of myself. Oh, I know I don't have the bloom that I had when I was 20. I don't look like I did when I was 22. I have to face the fact that I'm getting older. In my mind, I'm 26! But men don't look at me and see a 26-year-old girl. I'm beginning to accept that [laughs]. I'm beginning to accept the aging process.

A few years after her mastectomy, Wanda's mother's health began to fail. Wanda began returning to her hometown on weekends to stay with her mother. Later, she began to hire companions to stay with her mother during the week.

But it got to the point where I couldn't handle the companions from another city. And things were coming to a point where even with the companion's help, it wasn't going to work. So I moved back, because I knew it was getting to that stage. I wasn't happy to come back. I was just a good daughter, and I stood by her in her old age.

Wanda reported that her brother was no help with their mother—he had the "typical" attitude of "Let the sister do it," and "I did it." Although Wanda did not live with her mother, she assumed full responsibility.

I just did everything. I did the grocery shopping. I got the medicine. Took her to the doctor. I was getting very close to her though all this. Really very close. I couldn't have gone through the rest of my life feeling that I didn't help her handling the end of her life. So that part of the feeling is good.

Wanda felt very satisfied that she was able to provide this care for the woman who raised her. She knows that she "did the right thing." Furthermore, her mother was very appreciative—"She was not complaining or unpleasant. She was just so appreciative. A very tender thing, she was."

Since her mother's death, Wanda has felt somewhat isolated.

As a single person, I'm not connected to anything. You know, before my mother died, the connection was there. When you're looking after a parent, it's just like looking after a husband or a child. So I don't have that connectedness of "looking after" any longer.

At this point, Wanda is not sure where her life is going. She is not really happy living in her hometown. She had planned to get involved in local organizations but has only been marginally involved in the Reach to Recovery program. She does feel that her experience with breast cancer has had a good side.

That is the one good thing that comes out of it. You never complain over the little things any more. Life is so precious and so beautiful to you. I don't want to sound like a Pollyanna, but I am just so happy to see that tree out there, or to have a good meal. Everything is intensified. If you hadn't had that operation, you'd go around and complain if you had a hangnail, or if your hem is falling out. I have learned something since my operation. I found out in life, there is trouble, and there are problems. Trouble is when you have a mammogram, and the doctor says, "Come on in!" Problems are when you lock yourself out of your apartment, or you get stuck in traffic. Problems never worry me anymore. *Nothing* bothers me anymore if it's in the problem category. Things just don't get you down, because you have that inside feeling of "Thank God I'm alive!" You know that life is a gift. What a gift!

CASE 3: GWEN

Gwen, at age 59, had been a teacher for many, many years. She was single and lived with an old friend. She had no family in the area, although she did have a mother (age 93), and several sisters and brothers. She was the youngest child in the family. She decided to retire from her job, because it had become too demanding. "I really felt burned out from teaching." One month later, she was diagnosed with breast cancer.

I had discovered a lump 2 years before. It was external. It was just a real tiny lump, and I went to the gynecologist, who said it was not cancer. So I was relieved, really relieved. I had been just terrified! So then, I forgot about it. Then, 6 months later, the lump seemed to have changed to me. It really became more defined. I went back to him [the gynecologist], and he said, "no," it was just the structure of my breast. He said I had fibrous cysts. But then in May of last year, I thought, "Now the lump is really changing. The skin is beginning to dimple." I thought, "I've got to go back to him." So I went back. At this point, I had stopped going to doctors unless I had to, because of money. He still said it wasn't cancer, so I suggested we try a mammogram, and he said, "Sure." I was in no hurry, so I made an appointment for 3 weeks later. They called me the day after the mammogram and said to come back in for more pictures. It seemed ominous to me. But I was still optimistic it wasn't cancer. Then the gynecologist called me and told me that it looked cancerous. I was *so scared*, knowing that I'd had it for 2½ years! Within a half hour, I was in a surgeon's office, and he was examining me. He said he thought I had cancer in the third stage. I didn't know what that meant, and I was too scared to ask, but I knew it was bad. He was very pessimistic. He came into the waiting room, where he told my friend, "It's very serious. Shall we call her family?" Then he put his arm on her shoulder, as though to comfort her. That was his attitude. Very pessimistic. I stopped going to him for follow-up visits as soon after the surgery as I could.

Two days later, Gwen had a modified radical mastectomy.

The day of the surgery was the worst day in the world. It was raining so hard. That morning, I was going through my financial affairs, thinking "I'm probably about on the way out, so I'd better get things straightened out." I also called a minister to come over to see me, which was super! He really was quite a help. Then I got to the hospital, and there was a mix-up in the schedule. So the surgeon says to me, he says, "Nothing's gone right today!" Then in the surgery, he couldn't find any of the lymph nodes. Later, he was very apologetic. He really was embarrassed that he couldn't find the lymph nodes. But the surgery itself was really not that difficult.

Gwen received support from many friends after her surgery, and has learned from this how to better help others who are ill.

I got more cards and more flowers than I could ever imagine in my whole life. That was really supportive. It really matters. Now, when people get ill, I can recognize in a new way what it means. I can do things for them. I sure appreciated what people did for me. It's been the most wonderful gift for me to be aware of how other people experience illness. I have a friend who died of cancer before I had the breast cancer. I could hardly bear to go visit her. I feel guilty about that. Now, I feel like I can sort of make it up to other people what I didn't do for her. Because now I'm not afraid. I'm simply not afraid. I'm not afraid of death. If it comes, or when it comes, it comes. There's a way to help people. Being there is one way—just allowing yourself to be there. Just tolerate the discomfort, and be there.

Although her friends were supportive, having cancer has changed Gwen's friendship patterns.

I had this one friend who was pretty close. I do think that she really pulled back from the cancer. I have some other friends who I used to see a lot, and I see them much less now. They're retired, and they like to go around and have fun. That isn't my style. I'd rather do something that seems more fulfilling to me. And socially, we used to talk about things that didn't matter at all. Now, I'm talking with my friends on a level that matters. It's nice to be on a level where you can talk about life and death.

After her surgery, the laboratory reports showed that the tumor was receptive to hormones, and hormone-blocking treatment was recommended. Gwen went to a large cancer center at a teaching hospital to have a second opinion. Here, a lump was discovered under her arm, and a second surgery was done to remove this and the lymph nodes that were missed at the mastectomy. Luckily, none of the lymph nodes found were positive. Radiation therapy was recommended in addition to the hormonal therapy, however.

I started radiation the end of March, and it went until early May. And that's a daily affair. Radiation was harder for me than most women. For one thing, I was scared by the machine. Like I have a phobia. It's real big, and it makes a terrible noise. They leave you there, and they say, "Don't move!" I guess it's the fear of what the machine's doing to your body, because it is pretty powerful, and they are pretty specific about what they're trying to hit. By the second day, it was almost more than I could stand. I was praying, and the prayers weren't helping. My friend suggested that I pray for what to pray for, since my prayers didn't have a focus. I did that, and the answer was to pray for the technicians. So, when I did that, all my fear left me absolutely. But I still found it very tiring.

Gwen takes tamoxifen, an estrogen blocker.

There are a lot of side effects. The ones I have are getting too hot or too cold—icy cold—which is aggravating. I also have a yellow discharge. And sometimes I worry about taking a very strong medicine on a daily basis. I wonder what's happening to my system. If it attacks the cancer, then what else does it attack?

Gwen is not happy with her body image following the mastectomy, but she is not interested in reconstruction. Instead, she feels that accepting her body as it is now is just another part of aging.

I didn't have time before my surgery to mourn for my breast, like some people do. Because of the speed with which I had my surgery and the worry about my life, I didn't even think about the breast and what it was going to be like. So I went into a sorrowful period that I hadn't said "good-bye" to my breast. I think I'm beginning to feel a little less disgust at my body. The way our bathroom is set up, we have this great big mirror, and when I get out of the shower, there I am. I'm so lopsided. I think, "It's so ugly." I feel sort of angry about it. But I feel less of that than other women, not having a sexual relationship with anyone. But it still doesn't seem right to me. And it's a pain in the neck to always have to wear a prosthesis. An aggravation. I went to a wonderful meeting at the American Cancer Society on prostheses. The woman who gave the talk was real *big busted*, and she wore a real tight sweater, and it was clear that people couldn't tell which side had the prosthesis. It was very impressive.

I'm not considering reconstruction at this point. As you get older, your body begins to fall apart in different ways, and so it seemed like one more way. I don't find getting older easy at all. I didn't have to wear glasses until I was 50. That's just the biggest bother. Then, not too long ago, I got a hearing aid. It was hard for me to decide to do that. It was sort of like giving in to something. For me, the thing is not to be upset about it, and just let it go. So the breast just sort of fits in with that. I just need to let it go. It's just another situation that you can't control about your body.

Gwen did a variety of things to help her cope with her cancer experience. She read several books, which convinced her that she could beat the cancer. She began meditating. She took courses and workshops. She also attended support groups.

I started right away going to some support groups, which is unusual. It usually takes more time to digest the experience before you are ready to go and listen to other people's. A lot of people can't stand to hear about it right away. In fact, I didn't even want to go at first. I had to take myself in hand, and say, "Well, you're going to go!"

Eventually, Gwen became a co-leader of one of the support groups. She felt that her recovery was progressing well when, 6 months after the radiation ended, she began having pains in her chest.

They took a chest x-ray, and there was a spot on my shoulder. So then I spent that whole weekend absolutely convinced that I had cancer again. That sort of opened the floodgates for more fears. I guess I used denial after the surgery. I decided I was going to make it, and then I tried to put it all behind me. I just think I had stuffed enough of it down that it just had to come up. Even after they found out that the spot on the x-ray wasn't cancer, the fears kept coming up. Every time I experience pain somewhere in my body, I think, "It's probably cancer" again. So then I started seeing a psychologist. That proved to be very helpful, because I just talked my way through a whole lot of fears and a whole lot of anger.

From her reading, Gwen believes that people who get cancer have had difficulty expressing anger.

That would certainly be me. I don't have trouble in being angry for a lot of different things, but when it comes to meeting my own needs, sometimes I don't even sense the anger, or, if I sense it, I don't do anything about it.

Gwen has been working on changing her goals in life and her need to be in control.

The issue of my life has always been one of control—wanting to be in control. Cancer really throws you out of control, for sure! But then you realize that there are things you can control—your energy, for example. I'm learning to think that when something doesn't work out as I wanted it to, that's not necessarily bad. It just wasn't right for me. It's like a redirection. Like if I push in a certain direction and the doors are open, then I think, "OK, that's where I'm supposed to be going." But if the doors are shut, then I think, "No, that isn't where I'm supposed to go." Bernie Siegel (1986) says it's not that you need to have living as your aim. You can have peace of mind as your aim. That's something you can achieve if you work on it.

Cancer really hits you with: What's it all about? I was already struggling with this issue when I got the diagnosis. What am I supposed to be doing with my life? How do I pull it together? How do I ensure that I have activities which are really satisfying? The cancer helped me in terms of some of these questions. It increases your thoughts about what life is about. Is this the end of it? Or, if I do have more time, what is the most valuable way to spend that time? One of the books I read said that in 10 years, 55% of the breast cancer patients will be alive. It did make me think. Sort of gulp and think. I don't think I'm going to get cancer again. I think I'm well. But sometimes I do think

I have cancer. I know that if I did get cancer again, I would cope with it. They have wonderful medicines, and wonderful people, and wonderful ways of coping. And that's exactly what I would do.

Gwen has found meaningful things to do, many focused around her experience with cancer. As mentioned before, she is a co-leader of a support group. She also volunteers as a hospice worker. She has organized workshops for women and has spoken to many groups on healing. Gwen finds that she receives as much support as she gives through these activities. Thus, cancer has provided her with not only a network of friends but also a new meaning in life.

I do think that I enjoy life more now. Life is very good. To stop and appreciate it is great. One of the things I've been working on personally is really trying to find value in just being, rather than always doing. It's not something that I've mastered. It is one of my life goals now. Just to be content with the way life is now. Make each day count.

THEMES OF MIDLIFE WOMEN WITH BREAST CANCER: PART TWO

The case studies of Diane, Wanda, and Gwen are now used as a springboard for further discussion of important issues facing midlife women with breast cancer. The issues of confronting death, reassessing one's life, self-reliance, generativity, relationships with mothers, and friendships are further developed in this section. We focus on these issues and how they intersect with the breast cancer tasks of managing psychological reactions (anger and self-absorption), dealing with an uncertain future, and adjusting to role shifts. To develop these issues more fully, excerpts are included from the case histories of Sandra and Jessica (case studies in chapter 4) as well as quotations from Audrey (age 40), Sarah (age 42), Barbara (age 43), Clara (age 52), Ethel (age 53), and Marian (age 56).

Confronting Death

Researchers and writers concerned with issues of middle adulthood (Erikson, 1980; Gould, 1978; Levinson et al., 1978; Lifton, 1979; Neugarten, 1975) generally agree that in midlife the idea of death becomes more personalized as the adult faces the fact that he or she has probably lived more years in the past than he or she will live in the future. During the 40s there is a heightened feeling that "whatever we are going to do we must do now." The press of time is heavy as a woman comes to grips with the fact that she has lived at least one half of her life.

Diane, who was diagnosed with inflammatory breast cancer and given a little more than 2 years to live, found "the way they juggle time and statistics" to be "very frightening." By the end of the first year of chemotherapy, Diane was very sick and decided to take control of her treatment. She refused to continue with the 6 additional months of chemotherapy her doctor recommended. "I'm done; I will not continue chemotherapy. . . ." Instead, Diane used alternative treatments such as vitamins, visual imaging, massage therapy, and natural healing. Three years postdiagnosis she feels "it was absolutely the right decision." Diane, like so many of the women we interviewed, can't read an article or watch a television show without it triggering the fact that "I'm still very much at risk." She uses a combination of denial and positive thinking to cope with the issue of her own death.

Gwen came to terms with her fear of dying when she thought she had a recurrence 1 year after the initial diagnosis ("Every time I experience pain somewhere in my body, I think, 'It's probably cancer' "). Following psychotherapy, Gwen says, "Now I'm not afraid of death, I'm just simply not afraid. And that if it comes, or when it comes, it comes."

For Sandra (chapter 4) the task of coping with an uncertain future heightened her awareness of her own mortality. Dealing with this at age 40 may have intensified the rage and depression that she experienced after her diagnosis and treatment for breast cancer.

Barbara, diagnosed at age 43, expressed her fear that the cancer would return, and she "really hadn't been cured." Barbara feels as time has passed she has been able to accept the fact "that I might die." The way she came to accept it was to say the following.

> "Okay, I'm going to give it to You, God, and You're going to do whatever You see fit, and I'll accept whatever comes along." And that's the only way you get any peace.

Barbara had remarried before her breast cancer and found that her husband had more difficulty facing the possibility of her death than she did. Some research (Gotay, 1984) suggests that a husband of a woman with breast cancer is more likely to be disturbed by the possibility his wife may die than she is.

Barbara wanted a chance to talk about the possibility of her death with her family, to tie up loose ends, but her husband would not allow her to talk about it—"he felt like I was thinking negatively."

> The one area that I found the most difficult is that you feel that you're dealing with death and dying, and you want to talk about it—you should really have that liberty. You know everyone wants you to think positively, but there are times when you really want to talk about the fact that maybe you're not going to be here a year from now. Perhaps you have some possessions that are near

and dear to you, and you want to be sure that certain people get them, or you have things that haven't been said to someone, and you have all those loose ends that you feel you want to tie up.

Barbara believes that her confrontation with her own mortality as a result of her experience with breast cancer is "almost a good process" because it has made her believe that she could cope with any life-threatening illness. However, she feels she would have coped more effectively if her family had been able to listen to her concerns. It seems important that families allow the woman to discuss her concerns about possible death and try to understand that it does not make the patient feel worse, as Barbara's husband believed.

For Sandra, Gwen, and Barbara, the illness task of dealing with an uncertain future and the midlife task of confronting death have intersected in a positive way to further personal growth—but not without feelings of anger, depression, and resentment.

Reassessing One's Life

Midlife is thought to be a time of deep self-renewal when a woman may struggle to become the "adult self" she has been working on for many years (Gould, 1978). Midlife is often a time of reassessment and of reordering one's goals. "With the right attitude, this time period can become a time of reappraisal, renewed commitment, and growth" (Zastrow & Kirst-Ashman, 1987, p. 297). Neugarten (1975) and Gould (1978) speak of midlife as a time of "stock taking" when adults try to assess how their lives are going to turn out. This takes into consideration one's external achievements as well as concerns about inner satisfaction and the "hope of achieving a sense of completion and fulfillment" (Lidz, 1980, p. 29).

According to Young-Eisendrath (1984), middle-aged adults must develop a capacity to tolerate their shortcomings—to integrate their own sense of vulnerability and weakness into their self-image. The ability to begin to move in this direction can push the middle-aged woman toward internal growth. The need to grapple with loss and limitation as part of one's sense of identity comes into sharper focus for a woman threatened with the loss of a breast.

All women diagnosed with breast cancer have to come to grips with the fact that they have an uncertain future. Almost all of the women we interviewed, regardless of age, responded to this challenge by reassessing their lives and refocusing their priorities. Ultimately, these women learned to "make every day count" and to live their lives to the fullest. There is a close correspondence between this process and the type of reappraisal that is common in midlife. Because many midlife women were already going through this process, this piece of the breast cancer experience was especially salient for them.

Diane was in her mid-40s when she reassessed her life because "I was about to lose the most important part of my extended biological family." Diane was the primary caregiver for three relatives who were critically ill and soon after these relatives died, she was diagnosed with breast cancer. Diane's breast cancer forced her to reassess her life again, and this time she changed the way she was living "in very fundamental ways" ("I knew I had to start living in the present"). Diane believes that "I'm a totally different woman than I would have been if you'd talked to me 5 years ago." This is an example of the reassessment that comes with midlife and the self-absorption that follows an experience with breast cancer intersecting to promote personal growth. Diane sees cancer as a "remarkable opportunity to make it a growth experience if someones chooses to use it that way."

Gwen claims that her semiretirement coincided with midlife reassessment and breast cancer (dealing with an uncertain future) to promote personal growth for her. She believes that the cancer experience helped her ask herself important questions like "What am I supposed to be doing with my life? If I have more time, what is a valuable way to spend that time?" Directly as a result of her experience with breast cancer, Gwen is learning to trust the ebb and flow of life—the process of living. She is learning to "just let go of the control," and if she pushes in a "certain direction and the doors are open" then she knows that's where "I'm supposed to be going."

Sandra (chapter 4) was 40 years old and at the beginning of midlife when she was diagnosed with breast cancer. She went through a period of deep depression and even considered suicide, but has used the 10 years following her surgeries to struggle with integrating her new body image and her new self-awareness. This is the internal growth that Sandra describes when she says, "I came out of the other end a different person. It's just amazing, I came to several realizations, and it seems the older I get the more I think about it. I mean, every other month there's a new revelation. I'm not afraid to stand on my own two feet. I feel pretty good about myself."

At midlife, reassessment intersects with the breast cancer tasks of self-absorption and facing an uncertain future. These tasks can help a woman to reexamine and reappraise her life on an even deeper level than she might do in the ordinary midlife "stock taking." Certainly the sense of urgency felt in midlife is heightened by breast cancer. Unlike early adulthood, when self-absorption can increase the risk of not achieving a sense of intimacy, in midlife it can intersect positively with the life-phase task of reassessment to promote personal growth.

Self-Reliance

The growing literature on female adult development indicates a tendency for midlife women to move toward autonomy, self-reliance, and in-dependence (Norman & Scaramella, 1980; Rubin, 1979). Perhaps this comes as a result of the reassessment discussed in the previous section.

Reinke et al. (1985) found that at midlife women become more assertive and autonomous. "Middle aged women exhibit increased assertiveness, dominance, achievement orientation, increased involvement in the sociopolitical world and the work force, and, finally, increased psychological well being" (Reinke et al., 1985, p. 1354). Rubin (1979) found that women in midlife (who have spent their earlier years nurturing families) desire "achievement, mastery, competence—the desire to do something for themselves" (p. 25). Colarussa and Nemiroff (1981) report additional findings that confirm Carl Jung's (1933) observation that as women age they "become more comfortable with their aggressive and assertive impulses, while men develop greater acceptance of their nurturing and affiliative impulses" (p. 51).

Since struggling with breast cancer, Diane has learned to take better care of herself by taking more vacations and by planning her social schedule ahead of her work schedule. Diane says, "That would never *ever, ever* have happened if this [cancer] had not happened." Another woman we interviewed had a similar reaction.

> You've got to take care of yourself. So I made a little program for myself; I was going to take breaks—I was going to try to get better all year. I was going to cut out some of the evening activities that I had gone on, and just little by little I guess I regained strength again, and gradually, I came back to myself.

Coping with breast cancer often brings with it reflection and self-absorption. Because of increased self-observation, Gwen says, "I'm really aware of a lot more negatives in my life than I was before." Gwen says she copes with anger better since her experience with breast cancer. This anger is specifically related to meeting her own needs ("When it came to meeting my own needs, sometimes I didn't sense the anger, or if I sensed it I didn't do anything with it"). Gwen has also worked at getting more support in her life and seeking more meaningful relationships.

Following her experience with cancer, Sandra learned to take care of herself after years of focusing on the needs of others ("I'm not afraid to stand on my own two feet"). After Sandra and Beth (chapter 4) dealt with the immediate crisis by helping their husbands, children, family, and friends cope with their disease, there seemed to be a need to turn inward for stamina and an "I can survive on my own" attitude. Sandra believes that her experience with breast cancer has changed her life dramatically.

Before her mastectomy, Sandra describes herself as having been a "pleaser—part of my existence was making everybody happy, but to the point where I worried about everyone else. I wasn't a happy person." Some time after her last breast reconstruction, Sandra realized that she needed to become more assertive and active regarding her own welfare. She now takes time out for walking, laughing with friends, and treating herself— instead of taking care of others at the expense of her own needs. "I'm learning to speak up for myself. And not be afraid of repercussions."

The self-confidence that women gain by observing their own success in coping with breast cancer and its treatments may help them to achieve the self-reliance for which many midlife women are striving. Although women who were diagnosed with breast cancer in their 20s have discussed a similar reaction (learning to say "no"), at midlife this new found self-reliance may have special meaning because of the impact of their confrontation with their own mortality and a sense of "less time to live."

Generativity

Midlife adults want to experience a personal sense of effectiveness and want "to make a difference" (Newman & Newman, 1987). Erikson (1980) reports that middle-aged adults experience a growing need to leave something behind for the next generation. If adults do not experience their sense of generativity they can be vulnerable to stagnation (Erikson, 1980). For women, this sense of generativity does not begin at midlife, because most have already invested in caregiving and relationships before this phase (Gilligan, 1982b). In findings from a survey of 1,200 middle-aged adults (men and women), most adults report that they perceived middle age as a time of "intense deepening of relationships and acts of caring" (Goleman, 1990). Both men and women indicated a deep concern for contributing to the well-being of society. These findings seem to support Erikson's assumption that generativity is the pivotal point of personal growth in midlife for both sexes.

An experience like breast cancer can help the midlife woman move toward generativity if she achieves a renewed confidence in herself and a reinvestment in people or activities outside the family following the period of reappraisal. At midlife, many adult women are confronting the loss of parents and of children who are often moving out of the home. Successful adaptation to this phase "requires emotional reinvestment in people or activities outside the family or sphere of close friends" (Blumberg et al., 1982, p. 9). If a woman cannot establish alternatives, this sense of loss may be magnified, creating a feeling of isolation that can be compounded by an experience with breast cancer (Blumberg et al., 1982), with its self-absorption and turning inward.

Before her diagnosis of breast cancer, Gwen had resigned from a teaching position that was sapping her energy ("I'd rather be doing something that is more fulfilling to me. . . . Cancer throws you out of control but then you realize that you can control your energy"). Instead of turning inward, Gwen has used her breast cancer experience to redirect her energy toward developing and leading workshops for women and is about to take on a part-time position as a counselor for teenagers at a school. "This is work that I enjoy; I enjoy the association."

Following her experience with breast cancer, Sandra (see case study in chapter 4) spoke of having to "make a commitment"—to decide what she wanted to do with the next 20 years. Her husband is at a point in his career when he has more flexibility and wants Sandra to do some traveling with him. She is in conflict because she wants to spend her time in a more meaningful way—contributing her talents to society. Sandra wants to achieve a sense of accomplishment outside of the home ("I have this commitment that is very important to me. I'm not very happy just filling my hours"). Her push toward generativity (that is part of a midlife experience) and the wish to make each day count (following her experience with breast cancer) have intersected to encourage Sandra to take on meaningful work.

Both Sandra and Beth (see case studies in chapter 4) committed themselves to helping other women with breast cancer. In fact, many of the midlife women we interviewed were highly invested in volunteer work with other women who had breast cancer. Others helped friends cope with breast cancer and other life-threatening illnesses. Diane said, "I know one of the things I legitimately have to give people now is a kind of experience that a lot of people don't have."

Some midlife women, however, had not yet been able to use their breast cancer experience to foster personal growth at the time of the interview. Wanda has not yet found a connection that would serve as an outlet for her midlife expression of generativity; thus, she runs the risk of emotional stagnation. Wanda admits that "this is the first time in my life I've ever said, 'it's flat.' I could be in trouble if I don't handle it right. It can be a downward spiral of depression, boredom, and all of that." At the moment her coping style is to find "perks" by taking trips to stimulating cities—"a week here and a week there."

Sylvia has been unhappily married for several years. Her four children are married, and she is experiencing loneliness, depression, and severe anxiety about the possible recurrence of breast cancer. At the age of 58, Sylvia has never learned to drive a car and has never worked outside the home. Although she would like to become employed, she is fearful of applying for a job because of ageism and her lack of marketable skills. She is considering doing some volunteer work that would be meaningful to her.

Another woman, diagnosed with breast cancer at age 43 and separated from her husband at that time, claimed that her experience with cancer resulted in her seeing a counselor who helped her to "discover herself" and to determine what she wanted to do with her life. Like Sylvia, she had never worked outside the home while she was married and had not developed marketable skills. Through counseling, she discovered she wanted to work in the helping professions and took a job as a nurse's aide in a nursing home. This midlife woman's experience with breast cancer seems to be one factor that enabled her to make a commitment to meaningful work. She further indicated that the volunteer work she does for Reach for Recovery "is the most rewarding thing in my life now." It seems that midlife women are looking for opportunities in which they can feel appreciated and experience visible evidence of personal effectiveness. The actual opportunities available to women can affect the degree to which their needs for commitment and generativity are satisfied.

Generativity, in the form of a reaching out to have an impact on the larger society, may be new for midlife women who had traditional marriages and had not developed careers that could have given them a sense of accomplishment. This life stage may be different for upcoming cohorts who have had challenging careers since young adulthood.

In terms of the breast cancer tasks, self-absorption (common in early adjustment to breast cancer) may be helpful in the reassessment stage but could hinder the woman who is focusing on generativity. Breast cancer may also provide women an opportunity for expressing a sense of generativity. The solution to the question of "what meaningful activity can I perform?" is answered because they can now reach out to other women with breast cancer in a way that others cannot. This may explain why so many of the volunteers in the American Cancer Society programs (and in our study) are midlife women.

Relationships with Mothers

During midlife, role shifts between the two older generations, which we saw begin in the 30s, are even more prominent, as the oldest generation becomes more dependent on the middle-aged generation—particularly the woman who is involved in caregiving (Brody, 1981, 1985; Brody, Johnson, & Fulcomer, 1984; Cantor, 1983). When the tables are turned and the adult daughter becomes seriously ill with breast cancer, the daughter may need her mother for support.

At the time of her diagnosis and resulting mastectomy, Wanda was single and living alone. She needed her mother, and her mother was able to respond to her need and take care of her. Both Wanda and her mother enjoyed this period ("I needed her, and she just enjoyed nurturing me"). Research (Bankoff, 1983; Brody, 1985; Fischer, 1986; Walter, 1988, 1989) has suggested that older women still enjoy and benefit from the role of mother, and midlife daughters still need their mothers to nurture them. A few years after her mastectomy, Wanda took care of her mother when she became seriously ill and felt very satisfied that she was able to provide this care.

In our study, however, Wanda was the exception, as most mother-daughter relationships at this stage were described as problematic or non-nurturing. Diane chose not to accept the support offered by her immediate family and relied on a large network of friends and a cousin. Gwen did not count on her mother who was 93 years of age and lived far away. Instead, her niece and close friends cared for her following surgery. Most of the other midlife women we interviewed whose mothers were still living did not perceive their mothers as a source of support at the time of their diagnosis and treatment.

Clara, a woman who was separated from her husband at the time of her diagnosis, did not receive the same support from her mother as Wanda did. Clara's mother visited with her for a short time following her mastectomy but it was not helpful.

> My mother is kind of senile, and she really didn't show any feelings to me or anything. She's a homebody. She was so glad when it was time to go home. . . . That's the only thing she really seemed to have on her mind, getting ready to go back home and get on with her life.

Clara felt rejected and said, "Momma, I can't believe you're ready to leave me behind that bad." Two years after the surgery, Clara was hurt to discover that her mother didn't even remember that Clara had had surgery. At midlife it is likely that a woman's parents will no longer be a source of comfort or support because of their own physical and emotional needs.

Audrey (age 40) whose mother had had breast cancer years before, became very protective toward her mother who was experiencing so much guilt about having passed cancer on to her. Audrey tried to help her 70-year-old mother cope with these reactions.

> My mother was more upset than I was. I mean, of course she blamed herself; she says, "I gave you this. This is my fault." "Mom, this isn't your fault—what you gave me was an example of how somebody lives after cancer surgery," I said. She went through it real well, and she just had a very positive outlook about the whole thing. I grew up with a woman [who] had come through this and did real well and was always positive about her health and her life. . . . I wanted to help her realize that.

Audrey was more focused on her mother's needs and relied very little on her mother for emotional support. Instead she turned toward her friends at work.

In Jessica's case (chapter 4) her mother had a serious illness at the time of Jessica's diagnosis with breast cancer. Jessica felt that, although her mother "did try to be supportive of me and brought me presents and things," her mother was unable to be emotionally supportive of her during her crisis. Instead Jessica felt that her mother had "a way of turning the focus of everything back to herself," expecting Jessica to give to her. Jessica wanted some emotional support from her mother—as a daughter she wanted to be nurtured by her mother. Perhaps her mother avoided responding to Jessica's problem because of her own guilt feelings about the possibility of having passed cancer through family genes. At this life stage we see the aging mothers feeling responsible for passing on cancer to her adult daughter, interfering with her capacity to love and nurture her daughter at a time when she needs it. This is a parallel to the guilt we saw expressed by women in their 30s toward their adolescent daughters.

Another midlife woman, Sarah (age 42), had a more complex interaction concerning guilt. She and her mother "didn't talk too much about it," but Sarah was very hurt by a comment her mother made after her surgery.

> I don't think she meant to say it in a way to hurt me. Because I was always small [breasted], she said, "Well, you were always small, so. . . ." She said it so that I shouldn't feel so bad, I think. But that's not what makes you feel better, the size. She was downplaying it. It really made an impression on me, but I didn't say anything to her about it.

At the time of Sarah's chemotherapy, her mother was dying from liver cancer, so it was "a very difficult time." Sarah felt guilty that she was unable to bring her mother to her home to care for her.

> It was very difficult at the end, because she was in the hospital and they couldn't keep her there. She wanted to go home, but my father [age 80] couldn't take care of her, and she had to go to a hospice. I felt bad about that, but there was nothing that could have been done.

Here is a case in which the role shifts necessitated by breast cancer and its treatment become problematic because the adult daughter cannot carry out her role as a caregiver to her mother in a time of great need. This can produce guilt in the adult daughter and may produce great anxiety in her parents. In Sarah's case, her mother's negative comment may well have been a result of this anxiety and her fear that Sarah would no longer be able to provide support to her.

The breast cancer task of adapting to role shifts intersects with the mother-daughter relationship in different ways, depending on the type of relationship these women have established with each other and on the health of the mother. From our interviews with midlife women it seems that, aside from Wanda, most women were not able to turn toward their mothers for support. This caused emotional pain for those women who wanted their mothers to support them. Compared with women in their 30s, midlife women seemed more comfortable accepting their dependency needs but were upset when support from mothers was unavailable. Furthermore, breast cancer can make it very difficult for some midlife women to be caregivers to their mothers, inducing guilt in adult daughters and anxiety in mothers.

Because research suggests that women who have never been mothers are "affected more strongly by relationships with their mothers than are women who have children" (Baruch et al., 1983, p. 197), it may be especially important for women without children to develop alternative networks of support when relationships with mothers are not available or viable. Diane and Gwen are examples of women who are not mothers and who did not have supportive relationships with their mothers during their crisis with breast cancer, but who were very adaptive in establishing support networks with friends and extended family members.

Friendships

Gilligan (1982a) asserts that women reach midlife with a psychological history different from men's and "make a different sense out of their experiences on the basis of their knowledge of human relationships" (Gilligan, 1982a, p. 111). Because women experience the "reality of connection" as a given rather than as "freely contracted" they have a different view of the possibilities that relationships provide for both growth and oppression. Reassessment at midlife for women may mean reassessment of interpersonal relationships with parents, husband, lover, children, and friends (Garner & Mercer, 1989).

Although friendship is an extremely important resource for women throughout the life cycle, "the importance of women's close female friendships diminishes from adolescence to early adulthood as they focus on finding a mate and establishing a marriage, and then increases throughout the rest of the life cycle" (Carter and McGoldrick, 1989, p. 60). In our interviews, it was the midlife woman who placed heaviest emphasis on friendships. Younger women may have had to forgo close friendships because of the excessive demands of family and career. In midlife, when her parents may have died or are unable to provide support, and when children are either adolescent or adult and she is "letting go," a woman may be likely to turn outward to friends for support during a medical crisis, such as breast cancer.

When she does this she takes a risk that she may not receive the support she wants and needs. In her interviews with breast cancer patients, Johnson (1987) found that midlife women experienced a variety of reactions from friends. Some friends were very supportive, some avoided the breast cancer patient, and some old friendships were strengthened by the woman's experience with breast cancer. Diane reported that some of her friendships deepened following her breast cancer, and some "just kind of stayed where they were." For Diane, many of her friends were like family to her. One of her friends who could not be with her at the hospital organized a network of support so that she was never alone, once she returned home from the hospital. Diane "had three old lovers who were incapable of relating at all" because they were unable to deal with the fact that she had a life-threatening disease. Diane reported that later these same three women became part of her close friendship network, however.

Although Gwen received support from many friends after her surgery ("I got more cards and flowers than I could ever imagine. . . . That was really supportive"), she also reported that some of her close friends "pulled back." For Gwen, having cancer changed her entire friendship pattern. She sees much less of some of her old friends who "like to go around and have fun. That isn't my style." Gwen prefers spending time with friends who talk about meaningful issues and will do things together that are more fulfilling to her. Through her volunteer work with cancer patients she has developed an expanded network of friends and a new meaning in life.

Other midlife women also reported closer friendships as a result of the common experience with breast cancer.

> I had a cousin who had lung cancer, and we had not been really close because she was older. Every single day I was in the hospital she called me. We renewed our friendship just because she had cancer. It was a big help to me because she could relate to what I was going through, even though it was a different kind of cancer. She gave me a lot of support.
>
> Ethel, 53

Sandra (see case study in chapter 4) reported that one of her friendships was strengthened by her own experience with breast cancer. Her friend had a mastectomy years before Sandra's, but "she had never discussed it with me." Once Sandra had her mastectomy, the two opened up to each other. This pattern of midlife women reaching out to others who have breast cancer (old friends and acquaintances or new friends) was apparent in the lives of many women. One difference between these women and younger women is simply, that being older, they are more likely to know other women with breast cancer.

Friendships did not always withstand the strain of the cancer diagnosis, however. Several midlife women offered explanations for why some friends resisted seeing them or speaking with them after their diagnosis of breast cancer. Two women (discussed in the previous chapter), Jessica and Marian, felt that people just cannot tune in to your problem because they haven't been through it or they "don't want to know." The same factor that brought women closer to others who had cancer can lead to withdrawal from those who have not.

Marian offered this explanation for the withdrawal of friends. "People who are not suffering this [breast cancer], either themselves or with a spouse or child, don't really tune in, because they can't really know what you feel." Marian remembers her own reaction to a former neighbor who had a mastectomy. At the time, Marian wrote a letter full of optimism and encouragement. Later, after Marian herself had a mastectomy, she wanted to know all the details of her friend's experience. "Now I know that while people are genuinely caring, I don't think they really want to hear all the nitty gritty."

Jessica reported that many of her friends did not keep in touch with her and did not want to know the details of her cancer experience because they were "protecting" themselves—"they don't want to think it can happen to them" (see Meyerowitz et al., 1988). Related to this issue is the "contagion factor." Jessica said, "[A friend] doesn't want to be around me anymore because she thinks that she might get cancer from me." Sandra reported that "one woman was so uncomfortable with this [cancer] that she really chose to stay away from me." Sarah (age 42) also mentioned that some friends withdraw from a relationship because they "think that you're going to die if you tell them that you had cancer. They look at you differently." Like most women with breast cancer, Sarah doesn't want to be treated or "looked at" differently.

Perhaps these women are describing some of the conflicts friends experience in reacting to women who have breast cancer—conflicts that result in barriers to the patient receiving much-needed support. Wortman and Dunkel-Schetter (1979) argue that a conflict develops in friendships between negative feelings about the disease and a belief that the appropriate behaviors to display when interacting with cancer patients are optimism and cheerfulness.

Although some of Jessica's friends were supportive, she is bitter and disappointed with those who were not ("I have one friend that I thought would be right with me. Never once did I see her, nor did she call me"). Jessica has never been able to talk to this very old friend about her disappointment and now describes their relationship as one of "occasional contact."

Sylvia (age 52) expressed disappointment about the reaction of her closest friend (whom she had known for more than 20 years "like a sister").

> I was there with her—I don't want to say, "I did this for you, and you should do this for me," 'cause that's not the way I do it. . . . But when her husband had a stroke I was with her. I was there for her, with her, with him, making meals and all that, and then when I had my breast surgery, I'll never forget it. I didn't see her for 2 days (after coming home from the hospital), and she didn't call me. To this day I've never confronted her with that. As close as we were, she was the only one that never offered to take me in for radiation.

It appears that some women experience anger toward their friends, but are reluctant to confront them. They simply withdraw from the relationship or make it a less meaningful one. Ethel (age 53), however, approached her disappointment with a friend in a very different way.

> I have a friend . . . she can't handle sickness in her own family. She doesn't want to talk to people who are sick. She has some sort of phobia about it. I was in the hospital the first time (Ethel has had two mastectomies), and she didn't call me for 3 days. I knew how she was, so after 3 days I called her, and I said, "How come you haven't called me?" and she started to cry. She said, "I didn't know what to say to you." I said, "What did you say to me before I came into the hospital?" She said, "Well, you were all right then." I said, "Well, I'm all right now. So you talk to me the same way. Nothing's changed. I'm still me." She said, "Are you sure you're all right?" She was crying. I said, "Why don't you come in to see me, then you'll know." So she did and after that it was fine.

Ethel realized that even though she didn't hear from her friend after the mastectomy, she still cared and was struggling with her own feelings. Ethel's confrontation with her friend paid off for her.

It is not surprising that friendships are especially important to midlife women, in part because of the loss of support from mothers discussed in the previous section. Friends can provide an excellent source of support following an experience with breast cancer. In many cases, women need to learn to ask their friends directly for the support they need instead of withdrawing in anger when friends do not respond in the way they believe that they should. As hard as they try to communicate their feelings to old friends, however, breast cancer patients may have to accept the loss of some friendships. Peters-Golden (1982) found that the lack of expected support from friends resulted in women experiencing a poorer adjustment to breast cancer.

SUMMARY

Midlife can be a time of transition—for the mother–daughter relationship, a woman's body image, friendship patterns, marriage, letting go of children, confrontation of one's mortality, and one's personal goals in life. These transitions interact with breast cancer tasks in a variety of ways.

From interviews with women at midlife, facing their own mortality often intersects with breast cancer patients' task of coping with an uncertain future to further personal growth, but not without feelings of anger, depression, and resentment. Some women need their families to discuss their concerns about possible death and to directly confront the issues they are facing.

In many ways, breast cancer seems to form a context for women to work on the midlife tasks of reassessment, self-reliance, and generativity. Although women of all ages with breast cancer deal with the fact that they have an uncertain future by reassessing their lives and refocusing their priorities, there is a close correspondence between this process and the type of reassessment that is common in midlife. In our interviews with midlife women, we found that the midlife tasks of accepting limitations and the cancer tasks (self-absorption and dealing with an uncertain future) can push a woman to reexamine and reassess her life on an even deeper level than she might do in the ordinary midlife "stocktaking."

Instead of continuing to care for others at their own expense, some midlife women were pleased that their experience with breast cancer helped them become more self-reliant, increasing their ability to take care of themselves, while continuing to invest emotionally in relationships with others. It is important for women coping with breast cancer to be direct about their personal needs, without neglecting the importance of their relationships with others.

Self-absorption, the task common to early adjustment to breast cancer, may be helpful in reassessing one's life but could hinder the woman who is focusing on generativity. Because many midlife women are facing the loss of important relationships (parents, children, husbands), if they are unable to establish alternatives, an experience like breast cancer can only compound the isolation they already feel. As a result, some women in our study were struggling with a sense of stagnation and frustration. Some women were able to resolve this struggle by using their breast cancer experience to make a difference by investing in volunteer work with cancer patients, by becoming involved with meaningful work outside the home, or by helping friends cope with breast cancer and other terminal illnesses.

At midlife, the mother–daughter relationship has often shifted into a pattern in which the elder mother has become more dependent on the daughter for emotional and physical support. When the midlife woman is adjusting to breast cancer and an increased need for support, difficulties arise when she turns to her mother for support and does not receive it. Furthermore, breast cancer can make it difficult for some midlife women to continue as caregivers to their mothers, inducing guilt in the adult daughter and anxiety in her mother. It may be especially important to encourage women to develop alternative networks of support, when relationships with mothers are not available or viable.

We found that friendships are especially important to midlife women, in part because of the loss of support from mothers and other relationships (children, husbands), which may be less available to them. Although friends can provide an excellent source of support following an experience with breast cancer, in many cases women need to learn to ask their friends directly for support instead of withdrawing when friends do not respond in the way they need or expect.

6 Experiencing Breast Cancer in Later Adulthood

The case studies of Emily, Judith, Linda, and Elizabeth are examples of how women in later adulthood experienced breast cancer. Emily, age 69 at diagnosis, an active community volunteer, married with adult children and several grandchildren, chose a modified radical mastectomy. One week following her mastectomy her daughter and granddaughter came to live with her. Judith, single all her life, was diagnosed at age 63 after her early retirement from her job with a major corporation. Judith had a modified radical mastectomy with chemotherapy. Linda, age 66, was widowed 6 months before her diagnosis. Linda's adult children provided support for her experience with a modified radical mastectomy. Elizabeth was age 58, single, and owned a successful business at the time of her radical mastectomy (done in the 1970s). At age 73, Elizabeth's cancer recurred. She began an extensive chemotherapy program and was urged to enter a life-care community where she met and married her current husband.

The case studies of these four women illustrate important themes that were important for women in later adulthood. Coping with losses is a common theme in the lives of the elderly. In addition to the loss of a breast, Judith retired from her job and lost both of her parents, Linda experienced the sudden loss of her husband, and Elizabeth lost her business through retirement. Emily, Judith, and Linda all used religion as one way of coping with their losses. During later adulthood, relationships with children continue to change. For Emily and Linda a complex set of relationships between mother and daughter emerged, with dependence and independence on both sides. Independence is extremely important to the generation that is now elderly, and many elderly are willing to experience great discomfort to avoid being dependent. Following her mastectomy, Emily was eager to resume her household functions, Linda insisted on going home alone, Elizabeth (because of her strong need for independence) had a difficult time asking for the help she needed, and Judith had difficulty seeking help for her panic attacks and depression. Struggling with depression and despair is another issue faced by the elderly. Judith has been fighting her depression, whereas Elizabeth is coming to terms with her possible death by making a will and getting her affairs in order. In this chapter, these themes (coping with losses, relationships with children, independence, and depression-despair) will be discussed as they intersect with the breast cancer tasks.

CASE 1: EMILY

Emily had raised three children, and at age 69, was living with her husband in a small town in rural Maryland. Her children all lived out of state, but she had a sister and a brother in the area. Her other brother had died several years before. Emily's daughter was experiencing a rocky time in her marriage, and was considering leaving her husband and returning home with her young daughter. Emily and her husband were trying to help her and provide support but found it difficult to do long distance. Right when her daughter finally decided to move back in with her parents, Emily's doctor found a suspicious spot on her mammogram.

> I didn't expect it. I was in good health and had always taken good care of myself. I didn't neglect going to the gynecologist or the internist every year. But this was the first mammogram I had ever had.

When the doctor called and asked, "Do you have a surgeon?" Emily knew she was in trouble. The needle aspiration biopsy that followed showed that surgery was necessary. Emily was given the choice of a lumpectomy with radiation or a modified radical mastectomy.

> The decision was entirely mine to make. My husband said, "This doesn't make one bit of difference to me. You do what you think is best. I love you no matter what the changes are in your body." This was the biggest hurdle, to make the right decision. And you know, they give you so little time. They give you the weekend!

Emily decided to go ahead with the mastectomy. She was concerned that, if positive lymph nodes were found, that she would have to have a mastectomy anyway, and she did not want to have to go through two surgeries. Her age, she feels, was also a factor in her decision.

> You want to make the best appearance possible to everyone, and your husband certainly most of all, but it isn't as if you're in your 20s, with a young body. It's very different. We've been married for 45 years. And certainly by this time, you've had a lot of changes.

At the mastectomy, the doctors found no lymph node involvement, and Emily was told she didn't need chemotherapy. A week after she came home from the hospital, her daughter and granddaughter arrived on the doorstep. This was a very stressful time for Emily. She appreciated her daughter being there, however, because the support she was able to get from her sons was of a different nature.

> They [her sons] came, but they aren't coming to talk with you. They ask, "Mom, how do you feel?" but they can't talk about breast cancer. When my daughter came home, she was also able to help me with the dressings. There was a lot of swelling in my arm, and I had these exercises to do. But she was very upset about her own situation and whether she had made the right decision. She needed me for support, and I needed support at the same time. This was the first time I needed her, because I've been very healthy. She was trying to deal with her own problems and with me needing her. So, I got most of my support from my husband, and I supported her.

In addition to her husband, Emily also received support from her faith. "I think that if you have a strong faith, whatever it may be, this helps you through it." Emily also received support from friends.

> I was surprised by how many people, like through church or other organizations, came up to me and gave me a hug and said, "Yes, I had this too. I'm sorry, but you'll be all right because this happened to me and look at me!" I never knew some of these people had it. They never mentioned it and always appeared to be in such good health. I didn't know so many people had been in the same boat. These people were not close friends, and did not become close friends, but there is a bond between you.
>
> I think that when you get to be my age, and many things happen to your friends, ill health or other situations, you do find a support group. I do have a lot of friends, and, as they say, friends are the buffer in life.

Emily made a good recovery from her surgery. She was very soon able to drive again and do her housework. This was very important to her, because it meant being independent. "I like being independent!" Her husband did some of the housework right after she came home, but he was eager to relinquish this responsibility to her. "He will do anything for me, like do the housework, even though he doesn't like it. But only to the point where I can do it again. He isn't going to baby me."

In addition to doing the housework and driving, Emily was able to resume playing tennis. "I thought, 'I'll never be able to get back there playing tennis again,' but you know? The next year, I was able to play with friends my own age. The kind of tennis we play isn't too difficult, but it's the exercise, getting out there to play, and throwing the ball up to hit it. I wouldn't have believed I could do it when at first I couldn't even reach up in the shower!"

A year after her mastectomy, Emily was found to have an unrelated cancer in her kidney. She had to have another operation, in which her uterus and one kidney were removed.

> I think that having had the cancer of the breast helped me accept the fact that I was going to have to go through surgery again. That I shouldn't get too upset about it because the other surgery had turned out all right. I think the breast cancer prepared me in a way for the other cancer. There is a mystique around cancer, but that experience helped me to have a positive attitude. I had survived one cancer experience, and I knew I could survive another. And I have coped with other things, like three generations living together, and I have managed fine.

The mastectomy has affected Emily's self-image.

> It was very hard to look in the mirror. That was very very difficult. I still don't like it [2 years later]. I just hurry and get dressed. I don't look 'til I get my bra on. I don't like my husband to see me that way either. Even though he says it makes no difference to him. And I know he means it. But it does to me.

Despite this, it has not interfered with her sexuality.

> I thought it would. I still am very much aware—when I'm making love—that there's no breast there. I just don't like my husband to put his hand there. If he touches my other breast, fine. When I was much younger, I thought that when somebody reached menopause, they didn't have intercourse. Until I became gradually older, I never thought your sex life goes on. Maybe not as frequently. Maybe there are some changes with that. But if you're in love, and you're happy, you do have a sex life. I have some friends in their late 70s, and they still have a sex life. I mean it just doesn't stop.

Like so many of the women in our study, Emily felt that her experience with breast cancer has affected the way she lives her life.

> I try to enjoy every day as much as I can. When I have the opportunity to do something, whether it's travel, or a new experience, I do it. And it makes you think twice about the things that are petty. There are just some things that aren't worth being angry about. You can get around a lot of things by being diplomatic. Sometimes you can just not answer. I hardly ever make an issue out of something unless it is very, very important. I just want to enjoy life and enjoy other people.

CASE 2: JUDITH

Judith, who has been single all her life, lived alone in a small apartment in Manhattan. After her father died from cancer, her mother came to live with her. Ten years later, her mother also got cancer, and Judith cared for her mother until her death. At that time, Judith was 54 years old.

My father died when he was 67. My father's death really brought my mortality home to me. I hadn't thought of it much until he died. I guess that's true for many people. He needed a lot of care, and mother and I took care of him. He was quite ill. He was in dreadful pain. The whole episode was frightening to me. Then, when my mother got sick, I took care of her. I remember when my mom died, it was a blessing for me to go back to work. It really was. When you are working, you are forced to think about other things. It helped an awful lot.

Although her work was helpful to Judith in the period of mourning following her mother's death, a year after her mother died she decided to take early retirement from her job with a major corporation.

I had worked there for 38 years—my entire working life. I had had a number of different jobs. At the end, it was getting demoralizing. There were lots of cuts in my department, and I was getting up there in age. You know they don't do things for older people as far as career advancement is concerned. Things were falling apart at the seams, and they were starting to hint broadly. So I took advantage of the early retirement program.

Judith did well with her retirement at first. She took some college courses, and was busy with outings to the theater and concerts.

I was fine until I got this blasted illness. Since I retired, I've had a whole series of health problems—arthritis, skin rashes, surgery on my eye. All this after I retired. So maybe I should have stayed at work, I'm not sure [laughs].

It was during this period, when she was age 62, that Judith's breast cancer developed.

For 4 years off and on, I had had a bloody discharge from my nipple. I went to the surgeon, and he did a couple of biopsies, and he said it was benign. He did say there were some suspicious cells, and we would have to keep an eye on it. Then he let 2 years go by before he ordered another mammogram! And it was during that period that things developed. When he took another mammogram, he said it looked suspicious. I went in for a surgical biopsy, and it was cancerous!

Judith felt a lot of anger at her surgeon at this point.

I was very angry with him. I was angry that he skipped a mammogram, when all indications were that it should have been done on an annual basis. It's funny, the faith you put in doctors. Just assuming that they know what they're doing all the time, and that they have your interests at heart. In reality, you're the only one that has your interests at heart.

Judith's anger was not only because the cancer had not been picked up despite the fact that she was being closely followed by a surgeon. She was also very disappointed in the way her surgeon told her the results of the biopsy ("It was more than a biopsy—it was more like a lumpectomy. They took a large section of the side of my breast off"). Judith was just waking up from the anesthesia when her surgeon came into her room in the hospital.

> I was even more angry about the way he told me. I mean, he was very offhanded. I was still very groggy from the anesthesia. I was very sick. I was throwing up a lot. And in this period, when I was still fuzzy from the anesthesia, he comes in and sits down on a chair and says, "Well, it was like we thought it was. It's cancer." And up he goes out of his chair and off he goes. Well, I've never had such fear in all my life. I was there by myself. I was fortunate that my roommate had company at the time. The company came over to me as soon as the doctor left, and she stayed with me for a long time. She held my hand and talked to me. It was surprising how much that helped. Later, I went back to the office to have the stitches removed, and that's when he said I'd have to have a modified radical mastectomy.

Not surprisingly, Judith had lost faith in her doctor, and she sought another opinion.

> Probably like a lot of women, I didn't want to lose my breast. And, the fear of having it metastasize was always there, too. Always. So I went to [a major cancer center] to see if indeed I needed the breast removal, or whether I could have a lumpectomy. They said they thought it would be better if I had the modified radical, so I did.

Judith found some solace from religion shortly before her mastectomy.

> Right before the surgery, there was a religious congregation of the "born again" type that I went to. It provided an awful lot of help for me. It brought peace of mind to me. The day of the surgery, I wasn't at all panicked or anything like that. Even when I saw the results of the surgery, while it was horrifying, I didn't have that awful anger. But somehow or another, that feeling didn't stay with me.

In addition to this religious experience, Judith sought support from a cousin, who had also had a mastectomy.

> I talked to other people, but my cousin had the exact same thing, and really, she's been my support in all of this. I can't say that about any other person. She knows what I've been through, because she's been there herself. We get together and commiserate with one another. It does seem to have brought us together.

Several lymph nodes were found to have cancer involvement, and chemotherapy was recommended. Judith had a difficult time with this treatment. She went by herself back and forth to the chemotherapy at a major cancer center.

It made me dreadfully tired. I can't describe my physical condition, but it was just awful. Then, I developed thromboses from the chemo, and I had to be hospitalized for that. My whole leg had a blood clot in it! Then, they found a spot on my bladder and thought that might be cancer. They had to take a biopsy. Of course, that threw me for a loop. Fortunately, the conclusion was that the chemotherapy was affecting my bladder, and that it was not another cancer. In the middle of all this, I got quite sick with a terrible cold, and, because my white count was down from the chemo, I couldn't fight it. It was miserable, and it hung on for at least 3 or 4 months. It was my worst time. It was really my worst time. I had some rough times with that medicine. I'm hoping that the good outweighs the bad. I'm hoping that's so!

Like all women who have had a mastectomy, Judith had to cope with a major change in body image.

I had a good surgeon. In retrospect, though, looking at the scar, it doesn't look like he was such a good surgeon. But I didn't have any complications. There was no infection. And I took physical therapy to increase the flexibility in my arm. There were no physical problems. The surgeon said I did real well as far as the surgery was concerned.

I had large breasts, and to see just one there, when I'm in the bath—even today, it's very difficult. It's a terrific shock to look in the mirror and see nothing there. Now, they're following a spot on the right breast that showed up on my last mammogram. So, if that has to come off too, I might wind up being part man and part woman! Even though I don't have a husband, I'm still a woman, and it has affected me. I'm thinking about looking into reconstruction. I don't know whether I should, because I'm getting older. I know a lot of women my age would say that. But that doesn't really make any difference for me.

During the period while she was undergoing chemotherapy, Judith began to have "panic attacks"—something she had never experienced before.

It was in that period that I began to develop panic attacks. The first time, I was in bed, and I woke up. My heart was racing. I was pouring perspiration. I thought I was having a heart attack! Chest pains . . . and I said, "Should I call 911, or what?" I didn't know what to do. In retrospect, now, it's almost funny, but then it was not at all funny. I was absolutely terrorized. I've had several panic attacks since then, and I've come close a few times too. I try to occupy my mind—do physical things, like taking walks and baking, and most of the time that helps. But those panic attacks come on without any reason. The panic attacks really scared me. I don't think hearing about the cancer was as bad as those attacks. I just felt like I was going to die! I get into these depressed moods. I don't know *what* brings on the panic attacks, but I think depression might.

I think that I haven't faced up to the fact that this thing can kill me yet. And probably that brings on a depression. I think my first brush with death was my father. And it's been in the back of my head ever since then. Of course, I'm getting older, and with this disease, I just wonder each time whether this is it. I just bought a car, and I wonder if this is my last car, you know? That kind of thinking.

Judith went to see a psychiatrist about the panic attacks, and was given a tape with a relaxation exercise. The psychiatrist also encouraged her to take a mild sedative, but she resisted this.

> I wanted to tough it out. At that time, I think I was taking about 15 pills, and I thought I would gag if I had to take one more pill. I thought I'd tough it out, but it didn't work. For me, "psychiatrist" is a no-no. In my mother's and father's generation, it was very definitely a sign of weakness. I came from a tough family. They didn't show their emotions. My father had a horrible death from cancer, and he never complained or anything. Mother was more dependent, but she was that way too. And I guess it rubbed off on me. The opinion of any psychiatrist wasn't worth anything as far as they were concerned.

Judith sought support from a couple of sources other than the psychiatrist but with only limited success. She attended the American Cancer Society "I Can Cope" lecture series, but the volunteer who approached her there turned around and walked off when Judith mentioned her panic attacks. She attended a support group but found that she had little in common with the other members, who were much younger than herself. She began talking to a clergyman she liked, but he was transferred soon afterward.

> He was the kind of clergyman that I needed. He wasn't one of those patronizing kinds—the kind who just says, "Everything's going to be fine!" That I can't stand! I need somebody who knows what the score is and talks a real honest game. The other clergymen there are good men, but they are in the traditional mode. That doesn't help me when I need real advice and help. I just don't have [enough] confidence in them to approach them about anything important to me. So that's my bad luck!

After her chemotherapy program ended, things began to look up for Judith physically, although she fears she may never return to her former state emotionally.

> After the chemo was over, my frame of mind got better. I had lost about 60% of my hair, and that, of course, came back. I got stronger. The tiredness sort of disappeared, although I can't say I'm the same person physically that I was. Of course, I'm getting older. I just don't sleep well at all. I don't have trouble going to sleep. It's just that in 2 to 3 hours, I wake up. Then, I'm awake for a long period of time. I used to have a lot of activities and travel. But ever since I've had cancer, a lot of things have changed. I used to like going to the

theater, and musical things, but even that's losing its interest for me. I'm withdrawing almost all the time. I don't go out too much anymore. I used to have friends too, but I have gradually left those friends behind. I'm not interested. I've withdrawn. And I don't seem to want to do anything about it. I fight it. I really do. I fight it, and yet it's a real battle.

CASE 3: LINDA

Linda, at age 66, was a recent widow. She had four grown children, with two daughters living in the area. She also had several grandchildren, one of whom had spina bifida—a severe birth defect. The birth of this child had been very difficult on Linda's husband. "It broke his heart."

> My husband had been having heart problems. Three arteries were blocked, and they said they would like to put the balloon in to unblock them. He died on the table while they were inserting the balloon! The artery burst, which we didn't expect, of course.

Shortly after her husband's death, while she was still in a state of shock, she felt some soreness in her chest. At first, she ignored it, thinking it was because she had been exercising.

> After a week or two, I thought, "It feels like a lump!" And I went in. He [the doctor] felt it, and he said he couldn't really feel anything. I guess I could feel it because it was in there, you know? He said, "We'll do a mammogram." And he sent me over, and then he told me there was a lump in there.

Linda found the biopsy very painful.

> He [the doctor] wanted a biopsy first. I wish they would outlaw that. I think it's the Dark Ages, is what it is! It's the worst thing I've ever experienced, and I've been in the hospital some 80 times! They said they'd have to put this wire in to pinpoint it. They took a long wire, and they started to put it in up here [pointing to the top of the breast]. I said, "The lump's under here [pointing to the bottom of the breast]!" And he took this long, skinny wire and started inserting it into the breast. They don't give you anything [anesthesia]. *Nothing at all.* And they push it down, and push, you know? And I think, "Am I really sitting here going through this? This is the worst thing I've ever had in my life!" The nurse said, "It doesn't do any good to give you a needle, because that would hurt as much as that wire." So they put the wire in and took a picture. They came back and said, "It's not in the right place. I'll have to put another one in." So they inserted another wire! They took pictures again, and he came back and said, "I'm going to have to put that in from here." From the bottom up—where I *told* him to begin with! So they put in another wire. Then they put me on the gurney, and all these wires are still sticking out of me. I said, "This is barbaric! This is from the Dark Ages!"

After the results of the biopsy were in, Linda's doctor told her that her lump was malignant, and she would need surgery. He told her to come into the office in a few days to discuss the options.

> He said, "You should have it operated on. You should do the whole thing— take everything out." Then he said, "If you want, you can bring your daughter down—bring one of the girls down—and we'll sit here and I'll explain it all to both of you." And I figure, *I'm* the one that has to decide on it. There's no sense in getting anybody else to sit and listen to all this. [My daughter] would have had to get a baby-sitter. [My other daughter] would have had to bring [the handicapped child]. They were already worried enough. I mean, they'd just lost their dad. So I told him [the doctor] I'd get back to him, and a couple of days later I called him and told him to go ahead and set it up.

Linda believes that she did not feel the full impact of the results, because it happened so soon after her husband's death.

> After my husband's just dying a couple of months before that, I think after that, nothing else was really that important. I still wasn't straightened out from that. I mean, I never will be, really. But I don't think it really affected me like it would have if I hadn't already gone through his death. I was in such a shock. I was already so low with that, that I don't think this really mattered.

Linda's children were her main source of support during her operation.

> My daughters were there. They were holding my hand and talking to me before I went in for the surgery. My son [out-of-state] told the cardinal in his parish to dedicate his mass that day for me. To know that I was going to be operated on while he was saying mass for me—that was wonderful. And I felt as if [husband] was with me. Between the two of them, I just said, "Let's go ahead and get it over with!" I didn't have any qualms about it, or any fears or anything.

Linda felt fortunate that she didn't need any radiation or chemotherapy. Following her surgery, Linda returned to her home.

> My daughter wanted to come home with me. I said, "No. I don't want anybody with me!" It all depends on who you are and what you are used to. I had had four children, and with children, you get used to doing things whether you can do them or not. Before I left the hospital, I was brushing my hair and doing all kinds of things. I came home, and I did all my housework. The only thing I wasn't allowed to do was to run the vacuum. Like I said, it didn't stop me from doing anything.

Linda did not experience any difficulty looking at her scar.

> I would rather not see that it [the breast] wasn't there. It looks funny—one side and not the other. It's sort of strange, but it doesn't really bother me. If I (were) younger, and if [my husband were] here, I would feel badly about it, but it doesn't bother me that much.

Linda now spends much of her time at home alone. She does not drive. She used to rely on her husband to get around, and since his death, she has had to rely on her daughters to take her places. Although she took a series of driving lessons after she recovered from surgery, she never built up enough confidence to try driving.

Linda continues to experience some pain, almost 2 years after her surgery. She worries that this may signify a return of her cancer.

> You're always sore. It's always sort of numb. I get like a burning feeling in different parts. I guess that's where they cut the nerves. And the ribs are rather sore most of the time. Not *pain*. Just a little soreness. When I have a spot that'd be sore or something, I'd be thinking. "Oh, I hope this isn't—" what it could be and all. And I worry about if they'd find out there was something else wrong. I went to the doctor a couple of times and he'd say, "No." He couldn't find anything. So I guess maybe it is all right. But still, you wonder.

Linda relies on her religion for support with these feelings. She has not been able to share her fears with her children.

> I say a lot of prayers. If I start to get down and worry about it, I just pray for a while. I couldn't really do anything like that [share her feelings] with them [her children], 'cause they would get upset. They don't want to hear. Like, "Nothing's going to happen" or, "Don't worry about it!" You sit at home and worry about these things—that things are going to happen, or things are going to get worse—and they say, "Just forget about it!" If I say anything about something, they get all upset. "I don't want to hear it. Don't talk about something like that!" Talking about anything that might have to do with me dying. I think a lot of people want to talk about it with somebody, and they want their children to hear, but the children are just frightened, I guess. My mom used to do it too. She used to say things like, "Well, I probably won't be around by then," and I'd say, "Don't talk like that! Don't even talk about it! There's nothing going to happen to you." I realize now that she needed to talk about it. I realize now that I've gotten to this age, a lot of things about my mother.

CASE 4: ELIZABETH

Fifteen years ago, Elizabeth, at age 58, was a single woman who had recently lost her job when her (Pittsburgh) company went out of business. She was just getting started in her own small business when she learned that she would need to have a biopsy for a lump in her breast. She waited 4 months when she had a vacation scheduled to go in for the surgery. "It was thought by my physician and others at the clinic that I just had a [benign] lump." This was in the 1970s, when the biopsy and mastectomy were performed at one time. This is what happened to Elizabeth. She went into the hospital expecting to have a lump removed and to be ready to go on vacation the next day. She woke up with a radical mastectomy.

> I woke up in the recovery room. I was not really with it. It was just like a big room with bodies lying around, and I just started screaming for the nurse. I wasn't even aware then that I'd been operated on! The nurse came, but she would not talk to me about it. She wanted to get the doctor. It was then that I realized that I'd had the operation. The doctor told me that it [the cancer] had been very small, and he was absolutely certain they'd gotten everything. It was his feeling that that was the right thing to do.

At this point, Elizabeth received support from a nurse who had had a mastectomy herself.

> She was very casual about things. She didn't even have a prosthesis. She just had something she'd made and stuck in there [laughs]. She was very helpful to me. She helped me to get some kind of common sense about this.

Elizabeth also received help from her family, and she called friends to help cover her business while she was away. Although she lived alone, she reports that "there were people around—people to carry me back and forth for doctor's appointments." Things soon got back to normal, although Elizabeth remembers some soreness and pain in her side, and pain when she tried to drive. She was back to work in 3 weeks and was playing tennis the next spring. "I was not inhibited to play. I never could throw the ball up as straight, but I never noticed anything else." She did not even tell people at her business what had happened to her.

Elizabeth had an active social life. She attended many parties and functions, but dated on a selective basis.

> I was not dating anyone regularly at the time. By that time in my life I was very selective [laughs]. I didn't go out just to go out. I was never that kind of person. Occasionally I would meet someone whom I liked enough to start seeing regularly. I think at that point, you meet fewer people who are that attractive. So it was only when I met someone that I really wanted to get to know that I dated. Whether it took a longer time after that [the mastectomy] I don't know. I think that if I had met someone very attractive 2 months after [the mastectomy], I probably would have started dating him. As far as what I did, other than my work, I continued to see the friends I'd seen before. I had a lot of people around who were very very nice to me. I was the same person after the operation. I didn't think I was disabled. My prognosis was good. It was just a matter of getting myself healthy again and being able to go, to do.

Now, 15 years later, Elizabeth is age 73, and her breast cancer has recurred. She attributes her cancer to life stresses. Before her first episode, she had lost her job and had to set up her own business. Before the second, she found herself in a difficult situation with her neighbors. They had teenaged boys who were wild when the parents were out of the house. They played loud music, held parties, and disturbed the neighborhood. Elizabeth had complained and even called the police a couple of times. In retaliation, the boys had harassed her and even threatened her with violence. She became afraid to leave the house. Elizabeth feels that this experience wore her out, and made her feel helpless.

> Many times over the year before I became ill again, I was very, very exhausted. Around Thanksgiving, I was having such pain! I had back pain, and I just went to bed. I talked with my doctor. I was being treated for respiratory illness. She [the doctor] thought maybe I had arthritis or osteoporosis. My mother had had pleurisy and there were sharp pains at times, so I thought it might be that. By December, I just went in without an appointment saying, "I just can't tolerate this any longer. It's just too much!"
>
> As soon as she [the doctor] started examining me, she ordered blood work. I guess within a few days I knew that I had cancer again, and it had probably metastasized. I had seven lesions. The three in my back were the worst. In the beginning, I was in intense pain. I thought I didn't want to get into an organized (cancer treatment) program. I went to a private oncologist who's way out in the country. It was a bad choice for many reasons. For example, in terms of knowing what I could and couldn't do. I'd go in to get the blood work, but the doctor didn't explain anything. I wanted someone more alert than I was. I felt the need to sit down and talk with someone at greater length about this type of cancer. I went a couple of months, and then I said, "This just isn't the right thing for me."

Elizabeth arranged to transfer her care to a major academic cancer center, where she has been "exceedingly comfortable."

> In the beginning, my prognosis was very poor. I pushed [the doctor] about how long I may live. I was alone. I hadn't done a thing about dying. I said I just had to know, so I could make plans if anything happened. Get a lawyer. And he finally said that a year, 2 years perhaps, was the usual time. My other doctor also said that it was hard to say exactly, but that people with cancer this extensive didn't usually live very long. So that was depressing. I really wasn't ready to die.

Elizabeth had some difficulty asking for the help she needed during this period, especially from people who were not in her family.

> It was very hard in the beginning for me to gather around the people I needed. I didn't mind asking my family, but I think in terms of the demands on other people, that was difficult. I've always been very independent. But it worked out somehow. The woman next door took me to the hospital a couple of times in emergencies. Other times I was able to get my family. It was hard, you know, to wake up in the middle of the night and be so sick, and know I had to get help.

Elizabeth's doctor suggested that she move somewhere where medical care would be available if she needed it. So she moved to a life-care community, near where her family lived.

> At first, I lived in a single cottage. It was perfect for me. There were trees all around the cottage. I could sit out there and be quiet, away from all the noise. They sent my meals over.

Elizabeth was put on a program of chemotherapy at the cancer center.

> I go up [to the cancer center] every Wednesday to get the intravenous. On that day I start taking Cytoxan at home. I continue for 2 weeks. Then, I go up the following Wednesday to get shot up there with the chemo again. The only problem I have is that my white cell count is low. I get tired. I still do more than I should, but I do try to rest. After I went on chemotherapy, I didn't have any pain anymore, and I began to feel better. I could relate to people more.

One of the people Elizabeth met at the life-care community was George, a widower.

> It was a very interesting experience. By that time I had no intention of getting married. Certainly not with my diagnosis. George's first wife had had cancer, and he took care of her. So he's been through a great deal. I had seen him in groups and in the dining room. One night, he asked me to have dinner with him. And we started talking. Everything we have done and so forth. In a place like this, people are varied. Some are very interesting, but not a great number of people had my particular life-style. George did. My reaction was, I would never want to complicate this man's life, and have him go through anything like what he had with his first wife again. At that point, I thought he very well could if he got involved with me. But he is someone who I can talk to, and I enjoy. I know he felt the same way. And I thought, "Heavens! He's in awful shape in terms of how he's spending his life now." He was still depressed. It had been 3 years since his wife's death. "Maybe I can help him get out of the rut he's in. At least pull himself together and become more active and lead a more normal life." So this kind of justified it for me [laughs] I guess.
>
> I would never at that point have thought of marrying him. Never. And I'm sure he didn't think of marrying me either. But after we got to know each other, we were not the least bit concerned. He was a different person than I had ever known. I've wondered if it is easier to know a widower than a divorced man. We just were not the least bit uncertain about it.

Before getting married, Elizabeth and George went to the cancer center to talk with the doctors.

> We wanted to talk with [the doctor]. So we did, and after we got his blessing, well we went ahead with it. The nurse said, "And we thought *we* were the reason you were getting better!" So the next week we went up to Pittsburgh and got married. Then we had a small reception for my family, his family, and a few friends. It's worked out very well. Now I've got four grandchildren! I've

told him I'm not sure how much that made me marry him! (All these older people here are so excited. We were the first couple that had ever gotten married here. They're all talking about us. All the ladies are crazy about him, you know!)

After their marriage, Elizabeth and George moved to a new unit in the life-care community, and set up house together. They have been very busy with the move and fixing up the new place. Their lives have only just begun to settle down.

THEMES OF WOMEN WITH BREAST CANCER IN LATER ADULTHOOD

The voices of Emily, Linda, Judith, and Elizabeth are used to describe more fully the issues facing older women with breast cancer. These issues include coping with losses, relationships with children, independence, and depression-despair. Throughout this section the interaction of these life-stage issues and the breast cancer tasks of adjusting to role shifts, self-absorption, learning to balance hope and despair, and dealing with an uncertain future are discussed. Additional quotations from Jill (age 62), Renee (age 62), Cheryl (age 64), Theresa (age 70), Jeanne (age 73) and Pat (age 79) are used for further explication.

Coping with Losses

Loss is a theme in the lives of most elderly. They face the loss of physical health, the loss of important roles (e.g., retirement, children leaving home) and the loss of friends and loved ones through deaths (Kahana & Kahana, 1982). Judith retired from her job and lost both of her parents. Linda had experienced the loss of her husband very suddenly. Elizabeth had lost her business through retirement. Breast cancer also includes losses. If a mastectomy is done, a part of the body is lost. The cancer may also represent a loss of beauty, a loss of sexual attractiveness, and a loss of health. Thus the breast cancer may be one in a series of losses. This can have both advantages and disadvantages for the elderly woman. If she has coped successfully with other losses, she may be better prepared to deal with the breast cancer. Emily, for example, talks about how her successful experience with breast cancer helped her to deal with having kidney cancer later. "I had survived one cancer experience, and I knew I could survive another." Linda, whose husband died only months before her cancer was discovered, found the cancer easier to deal with because, in comparison with the shock of her husband's death, it seemed less important. There is

also evidence that that women's ability to accept their positive achievements and frustrations (integrity) and to cope effectively increases with age
(Hubbs-Tait, 1989).

For a woman who has already coped with serious health problems,
breast cancer may not represent a major loss. Mary, for example, at age 64,
has diabetes, is wheelchair bound and has lost the use of one of her arms.
She was able to use the coping skills she had already developed to help her
adjust to having breast cancer. Another example is Jeanne, who was 73
years old when her breast cancer was discovered. Jeanne had a terminal
illness of the liver that was discovered when she was 62 years old. She was
told at the time that she had only 5 years to live.

> I was devastated that I even had such an illness, and he [the doctor] said to
> me, "Look, you can be perfectly healthy and walk out on the street, and a
> truck will hit you and there you go. So—I don't know how many years you
> have, but whatever you have, you use—make the most of it." I'm a very
> strong person. I had a lot of adversity in my youth, but I was a survivor. I
> never went down. I never let anything get me down. I always had a philoso-
> phy—there's always tomorrow, there's always tomorrow!

Here, Jeanne shows how skills she learned in earlier crises helped her cope
with breast cancer.

The disadvantage of having other losses is that a series of losses can
easily prove overwhelming. Research on life events (Kasl & Berkman,
1981; Rahe, 1972) has shown that the more life events experienced (e.g.,
death of a spouse, serious illness, retirement) and the more serious these
are, the more likely the individual is to experience mental or physical
health problems. This relationship has also been found for breast cancer
severity and recurrence (Cooper et al., 1989; Ramirez et al., 1989). It is
also thought that social support can serve as a kind of buffer to life stresses
(Cobb, 1976; Cohen & Syme, 1985) That is, people with a high level of
social support may avoid negative consequences, even in the presence of
multiple losses. Unfortunately for the elderly, many of the life events
commonly experienced involve a loss of social support as well as a stressful
event. For example, retirement can cut a person off from friends. Death of a
spouse may mean the loss of a major source of support. Serious illness may
make it difficult or impossible to continue social activities. Judith provides
a good example. She experienced the death of her mother, retirement, and
a series of health problems including breast cancer. She also has very little
social support. She is single and has no children. Her relationships with
friends have deteriorated since her illness. She did not receive support from
her doctor or from the psychiatrist she saw. Nor has she been able to form
new relationships based on her cancer experience. It is hardly surprising,
then, that Judith is experiencing anxiety and depression.

Thus, although experiencing losses is not uncommon for older women, this may have both advantages and disadvantages for those who develop breast cancer. If their previous experience has resulted in effective coping skills or a strong support network, they may be able to cope with cancer more easily than younger women. Conversely, previous losses can be overwhelming and leave a socially isolated woman less able to withstand the challenges of a cancer experience.

It has been found that older and young women tend to use different coping mechanisms. One coping mechanism older women use more often than younger women is religious faith (Griffith, 1983; McCrae, 1982). Although the elderly are less likely than younger people to participate in church activities, they are more likely to engage in personal religious activities, such as prayer (Ainlay & Smith, 1984). In another study (McCrae & Costa, 1986), faith was ranked as the most successful coping mechanism among older adults. Emily, Judith, and Linda all used religion to help them cope with breast cancer. Emily was actively involved in her church and has a "strong faith." Linda was helped by having a mass said during her surgery. She also uses prayer to cope with her fears of recurrence. Judith attended a religious retreat before her surgery and sought counseling afterward from her clergyman. Another older woman (age 64) used religion to help her choose between a lumpectomy and a mastectomy.

> What do I do? My husband and I talked about it. I also talked with my minister. Then I just sat and read my Bible. One night, I stayed up all night in my bedroom, reading my special verses, and I prayed. And in the morning, I had found an answer somehow. I don't know where it came from, but I had found it.

Another coping mechanism older women tend to use, according to the study by Griffin, is "ignoring the problem." Emily talks about how she doesn't like to make an issue of things unless they are "very, very important." Judith tries to live up to the ideal set by her father and "tough it out." Linda says from raising four children, she got used to doing things "whether you can do them or not." Perhaps Elizabeth's decision to get married, despite her poor prognosis, can also be seen as an example of "ignoring the problem." Jeanne, age 73, also used this coping mechanism effectively.

> I put it right out of my mind. I just don't think about it. That's the way I handle it. I postpone thinking about it, don't dwell on it. I just went right ahead with life.

Eleven months after her mastectomy, Jeanne took a 'round-the-world trip. "I didn't know a single soul there, and I am reserved, but I did very well!"

When dealing with breast cancer, the older woman may want to review how she has coped with previous losses. The experience of breast cancer is likely to be more difficult for a woman who has not experienced previous losses, or for one who has had a series of overwhelming losses without a strong support network. Although counselors may be more comfortable with coping techniques like ventilation and other types of talk therapy, they should not overlook the value of religion and "ignoring the problem" for this cohort of older women.

Relationships with Children

Literature on relationships between older people and their children suggests that when financial, physical, or mental health deteriorates in an older person, a role reversal often occurs in which the adult child becomes like a parent to his own parent (Fischer, 1986). This is most likely to occur when a spouse is not available to provide the care needed. Because older women are much less likely to have spouses than older men (only 20% of women older than age 75 are married), this type of role reversal is much more likely to be experienced by older women (U.S. Senate Special Committee on Aging, 1981). Because breast cancer is a serious illness and some of the treatments can be debilitating, a certain amount of dependence on children may result. Thus a diagnosis of breast cancer may contribute to a role reversal process in parent–child relationships. We would expect this to be most likely in the period before and after surgery, and in cases where chemotherapy is used, because it is likely to interfere with functioning during an extended period.

In the case examples of Emily and Linda, we see different patterns. When Emily was coming home after her mastectomy, her daughter had just gotten divorced and moved back with Emily and her husband. Emily's daughter wanted support from her mother at the same time Emily was experiencing her own crisis and wanted to lean on her daughter. In Fischer's terms (1986), Emily wanted to shift to a role reversal, but her daughter resisted this shift. She wanted to maintain a pretransitional relationship, so that she could continue to rely on her mother for support. In this case, the daughter's needs prevailed, and Emily turned to her husband for support.

In Linda's case, we see pressure for a role reversal coming from outside the relationship. Linda's doctor suggested that she bring her daughter(s) into the office to discuss Linda's treatment options. Linda thought that this would burden the daughters, and that it wasn't necessary because it was her decision to make. Thus she rejected the doctor's assumption of a role reversal. Linda's relationship with her daughters cannot be called pretransitional, however. Linda has become dependent on her daughters for transportation and for social stimulation since her husband's death. At the same time, she remains a major source of support to her daughters, one of whom often needs her to baby-sit with her handicapped child. Linda's dependency is partly self-imposed, in that she has taken driving lessons but doesn't have the confidence to drive. It is possible that Linda is using this "dependence" to increase her contact with her daughters. Thus we see a complex set of relationships between mother and daughters, with both dependence and independence on both sides.

Another example of a complex mother–daughter relationship involves Pat, a 79-year-old widow. After Pat's breast lump was found, she decided to have a mastectomy on her doctor's advice. But her daughter had a different attitude.

> I had great trust and faith in the doctors. Now my daughter would distrust. Right away, she wanted to question the doctors. She'd argue! Whereas I wouldn't. So she did most of the talking. She said, "Let's not get rid of this breast if we don't have to." She called this surgeon and that surgeon. I suspect that doctors don't like to be disturbed and questioned about their decisions. I accept what they recommend. I thought they knew their business and would do the best that they could. So I was relieved when my daughter finally agreed with me that the mastectomy should be done. And it was a good thing, because they found it had already spread to the lymph glands.

Here, we see a different kind of mother-daughter relationship. Pat feels herself competent to make important medical decisions in her own way (by relying on her doctor's opinions). Pat's daughter, however, clearly does not accept this. She feels it necessary for her to come and protect her mother from insensitive doctors. The daughter took on an active role in her mother's medical care, not because she was asked but on her own initiative. Pat was not grateful for this unasked for help.

Moving into a role reversal seems to be easier for daughters than it is for mothers (Schlesinger, Tobin, & Kulys, 1980; Troll, 1982). In *Linked Lives*, Fischer (1986) points out that only daughters talk about "role reversal." Mothers do not acknowledge that they become like children to their own daughters. Perhaps this is what we see here. From Pat's viewpoint, her daughter is interfering. Because we did not interview Pat's daughter, we can only guess that her perception would be of a role reversal. After the surgery, however, Pat is actively involved in helping her daughter out with cooking and child care, although her daughter won't "let" her drive alone. So perhaps this is more of a "mutual mothering" relationship.

Another situation of strain between parents, children, and doctors is represented by Renee, who is 62. Renee does not speak English. She moved to the U.S. 10 years ago with her husband, and she has stayed at home, helping her husband out with his business. Her son recently moved to the U.S. and when breast cancer was discovered, this son became Renee's link to the medical establishment. He accompanied her to all doctor visits and translated what the doctors told her. The problem here was that Renee suspected that her son was not translating all that was said, that he may have been glossing over the truth. She worries that he is not telling her the bad news. Her frustration cannot be resolved because she is dependent on her son to communicate with her doctors! (One wonders if there has been a pattern in this family to "protect" each other from harsh truths.) This provides yet another example of a situation in which the nature of the mother–child relationship is not clear-cut. Renee is dependent on her son, but she is not happy with this situation. She would prefer to be able to communicate with the doctors directly. She is afraid that she is being "protected"—something that she does not feel she needs.

We see here a variety of patterns in older women's relationships with their children. In some cases, the relationship remains pretransitional, even though the mother may wish for more support from her daughter. In others, a certain amount of role reversal occurs, but this may be accompanied by conflicting emotions. The mother may resent her daughter's intrusion into her affairs or become more dependent than she actually needs to be. It also seems that mothers and children may perceive these situations very differently. We found no cases in which a complete role reversal had occurred because of breast cancer. Research on the families of the elderly supports the notion that even though shifts may occur in the exchange of help, a great deal of reciprocity remains (Litwak, 1981; Walker, Pratt, Shin, & Jones, 1990).

Another problem for women who have become dependent on their children is that they may also come to rely on children for social interaction. Most children cannot meet certain needs their parents have, however. Women with breast cancer need to be able to talk openly about their thoughts and fears. They also need to be able to express emotions, such as anger and sadness. They also may want to talk practically about death, and make plans for wills, burial arrangements, and so forth. Children are often not good confidants for their parents, however. Linda expresses this very clearly when she says that her children don't want her to talk about dying ("They would get upset. They don't want to hear. They say, "Nothing is going to happen," and "Don't talk like that"). The adult children themselves are probably in a state of denial. They are not ready to face the possibility of the parent's death. Thus they cannot be good confidants for their parents on these issues. In fact, studies have shown that relationships between adult children and their parents are seldom intimate (Lowenthal & Robinson, 1976), and that older people wanted more emotional closeness from their children than the children wanted to provide (Kulys &

Tobin, 1980). It is not surprising, then, that women who depend on their children for social contacts have lower morale than those who interact with friends and neighbors (Bankoff, 1978; Bumagin & Hirn, 1982).

Thus, breast cancer may further complicate what are already complex relationships between women and their adult children. This is especially so when women become dependent on their children. In these cases, a struggle may result between the woman's need for support and the child's continuing need for support and nurturance from her mother. At the same time, the woman and her child may be struggling over who is in control of medical decisions, where each may feel that the other is not competent to make these decisions alone. Other problems develop when women come to rely heavily on children for social interaction. In these cases, women may be blocked from expressing thoughts and feelings their children can't handle. It is important for those women who are dependent on their children for social interaction to develop other social contacts with persons their own age, or to use professionals to explore areas that are not comfortable for their children. With breast cancer, the need for care may be temporary, and in some cases, it will be more psychological then physical. It is important that the level of dependence not be exaggerated or prolonged, despite children's needs to feel they are being responsible.

Independence

Independence is extremely important to the generation that is now elderly. Many elderly are willing to experience great discomfort and deprivation to avoid being dependent. It is not clear whether this is a characteristic of older persons or whether it is unique to the current generation of elderly. Certainly the experience of the Depression, which had a major impact on the early lives of those who are now elderly, placed a high value on independence. Even without the Depression, however, it is clear that self-reliance is a basic American value, and that reliance on others is stigmatizing. Atchley (1980) points out that "the high importance given to independence in American society is related to the way we expect 'dependents' to behave. Dependent people in our society are supposed to defer to their benefactors, to be externally grateful for what they receive, and to give up their rights to lead their own lives."

Although many older women were socialized to be dependent on their husbands, they were also socialized to give help to others rather than receive it. For example, Emily, who was a traditional homemaker, was eager to resume her household functions. Although her husband did the housework right after her surgery, she didn't want this to continue. ("I like being independent!") Both Emily and her husband saw her continued dependence as "babying her." Linda insisted on going home alone following her surgery. ("My daughter wanted to come home with me; I said, 'No!' I don't want anybody with me!") She was proud of her ability to return to normal quickly. ("It didn't stop me from doing anything!")

Clearly, this desire for independence can be a good thing, providing a strong motivating force for the return to normal functioning. It can also cause problems, however. In fact, the strong sense of independence can lead to an underuse of services (Shanas & Sussman, 1979). In Elizabeth's case, for example, it made it difficult for her to ask for help ("It was very hard . . . for me to gather around the people I needed. I've always been very independent"). In Judith's case, the problems caused by her strong need for independence were severer. Even when Judith began to have panic attacks and depression, she had ambivalent feelings about seeking help. Although she had one visit with a psychiatrist, she did not take the sedative he prescribed. Nor did she follow up on the referral the study interviewer provided to a clinical social worker. She mentioned how her father had had terrible pain before his death and "never complained." In her family, displaying emotions was a sign of weakness. She wanted to be able to "tough it out." Judith's case shows how placing a high value on dealing with problems independently can lead to a failure to seek help when it is needed.

It is well known that the elderly underuse mental health services (Beck & Pearson, 1989). One study of 30 women between 55 and 85 years old found that older women managed their mental health alone and did not seek professional help unless it was absolutely necessary (Kaas, 1987). This is despite the fact that treatment for depression (the commonest mental health problem in the elderly) is as effective for older as it is for younger persons (Holzer, Leaf, & Weissman, 1985). It is impossible to weigh the benefit of mental health treatment for someone like Judith. On the one hand, she is experiencing very discomforting symptoms that may very well be easily treatable. Conversely, seeking and using such treatment may be a serious blow to her self-esteem. Because many emotional problems get better eventually without treatment, Judith may be better off in the long run battling it out on her own. Although she may go through unnecessary pain, her sense of her independence will be intact.

Services need to be developed for older breast cancer patients that provide needed help without threatening self-esteem. Traditional modalities may not appeal to them. For example, support groups were popular with many younger women in our sample but not among the older women. Only one older woman we interviewed had a positive experience with a support group, and she was the organizer-leader of it. One woman (Jeanne) attended a support group and found it depressing. "I couldn't stand it! So many of the women were full of sympathy for themselves. This didn't give me any support at all! I am a very private person, and I didn't want to discuss it. I mean, I don't advertise it, and I don't make a big display about it. And I don't want any sympathy!" Another (Judith) also sought out a support group but attended only one session, complaining that the women attending were much younger than she. Theresa, who is 70 years old, rejected an offer to attend a support group by the hospital social worker. "She said, 'Maybe that's just what you need, to discuss this with other people.' And I said, 'Well, I've never had the feeling that I'm in this alone.'"

Depression and Despair

In Erikson's model of life course development (Erikson, 1978, 1980), the crisis for old age (60–75) is integrity versus despair. Integrity, according to Erikson, involves being able to look back over one's life and feel good about it—accepting both one's positive achievements and frustrations. The process of life review brings a sense of closure to life. The negative resolution, despair, arises when the older person cannot accept his or her life and is unable to face death. There is an anger that life has gone by without the individual being actively engaged in it. Now it is too late to relive it. For Newman and Newman, the developmental tasks of this age include "accepting one's life" and "developing a point of view about death" (Newman & Newman, 1987). There is support for both of these theories in research on the elderly. Folkman, Lazarus, Pimley, and Novacek (1987) found that both elderly men and women more frequently used coping patterns associated with integrity.

Depression is not uncommon in the elderly, especially in women (Beck & Pearson, 1989). It is related to "taking stock of oneself and feeling that one's life will not improve significantly, and that one has achieved most, if not all, of which one is capable of achieving" (Kahana & Kahana 1982, p. 155). Although disengagement theory is no longer popular, it seems that many elderly become increasingly self-absorbed and gradually disengage from the external world (Cumming & Henry, 1961; Neugarten & Gutmann, 1968). Also, the elderly have been found to think about death more than younger persons but to fear it less (Kalish, 1976).

The experience of breast cancer presents a woman with several tasks that are quite similar to the developmental tasks of older persons. Self-absorption is common for anyone following a serious illness, and it is also a major process for resolving the crisis of this life stage. Depression is another common reaction to breast cancer that is also a part of the crisis of the aged. The old must develop a viewpoint about death, and cancer patients must learn to face an uncertain future. Cancer patients must learn to balance hope and despair—another task encountered by the elderly.

Thus, there is a high correspondence between the developmental tasks an older woman may already be working on and the tasks that breast cancer brings. To the extent that a woman has already worked through the developmental crisis of aging, her tasks in coping with breast cancer may be made easier. Many of the older women in our sample appeared to be in this situation. Previous illness and losses had already generated a certain amount of life review, of coming to terms with possible death. Many of these women spoke very matter-of-factly about death—something that we did not find in younger women. Elizabeth, for example, wanted her doctor to tell her how long she would live, so that she could make a will and get her affairs in order. Other examples are provided by Theresa (age 70) and Jill (age 76), respectively

> I said to him [the doctor], "Now, after surgery, how much time are you going to give me? And he said, "How much time do you need?" I was referring to how much longer I'd have to live after surgery, OK? So I said, "I need at least a year." And he said, "At least a year?" And I said, "Yes, I've got to get my house in order. Everybody's got to get their house in order, don't they?" And he said, "Of course."

Jill had two mastectomies, 12 years apart followed by a heart attack.

> Why in the world I'm even here to tell the tale, I don't know. My whole family died, mother, father, grandfathers, aunts, and uncles before they were 70 with coronaries. I come from a long line of coronaries. Why this old ticker kept plugging, I don't know. You're put here, and you've got to make the best of it as long as you're allowed to be here. I want to stick around as long as I can, unless I would not be able to function, and then I'd like to go. . . . The cancer may come back at another site, or you may die of something entirely different. Frankly, my choice would be another heart attack. But, if it's not to be, it's not to be. I don't want life support things. I want to go when my time comes.

These women seem to have come to some acceptance of death. This does not mean that they have given up the fight, nor does it mean that they have not experienced depression. In fact, some of these women talk about fighting their way through recurrent depressions. Jill, quoted earlier, says the following.

> I get depressed once in a while. I'm a Gemini. Most of the time I'm fine. But it's only normal and natural to have periods when there's some despondency. And then you have to gather your forces together, and harness them again, and go along. I love life!

Jeanne, who is 73 years old and has far outlived the life expectancy her doctors had predicted for a liver disease, says the following.

I reacted just like a child. I was angry. How did it happen to me? That's how I felt. Unreasonably. And I was extremely depressed. But of course you have to learn to adjust and accept. What else can you do? You know, you either swim or you drown.

Judith is fighting her depression ("I fight it. I really do. I fight it, and yet it's a real battle"). Perhaps her social isolation means there is nothing in her life to brake the combination of the life tasks and the illness tasks. There is nothing to pull her back from the self-absorption and the introspection. The depression that results feels overwhelming to her. Another factor here may be Judith's age. She was only 63 years old when diagnosed with breast cancer, thus she had only just entered the period of later adulthood identified by Erikson. She may have been hit with the cancer at a point when she was just beginning to grapple with the psychosocial crises, and the breast cancer may have pushed her even farther toward the despair that is normally being worked through at this age. Thus we expect that Judith's depression will give way as a result of her struggle. (In fact, when Judith read her case study, she commented that she was surprised at how negative she had sounded and how much better things were for her 8 months later. She had regained her interest in friends and activities, and has returned to an active life.)

SUMMARY

In our interviews with women in later adulthood it was apparent that how the woman has coped with previous loss prepares her in some ways for coping with breast cancer. The experience of breast cancer can be expected to be more devastating to a woman who has not experienced previous loss or to one who has experienced a series of losses without a strong support network. Professionals may be more comfortable with coping techniques like ventilation and other types of talk therapy, but should not overlook the value of religion and "ignoring the problem" for older women.

Breast cancer may further complicate what are already complex relationships between women and their adult children. In later life when older women may need to become dependent on their adult children for support, a struggle may develop between the older woman's need for support and the adult child's continuing need for nurturance. This struggle is often exacerbated by a mother's unwillingness to acknowledge that she can become like a child to her daughters or sons. Other problems develop when women come to rely heavily on children for social interaction. Women may be blocked from expressing thoughts and feelings their children cannot handle. It is important for health practitioners to recognize these conflicts, and not to inadvertently reduce the independence or underestimate the competence of the older woman. Women who are dependent on their children for social interaction can be encouraged to develop other contacts with persons their own age.

During her struggle with breast cancer, the older woman's desire for independence can be a good thing, providing a strong motivating force for the return to normal functioning. It can also lead to underuse of needed service, however. It is important for health professionals to develop services that provide needed help without threatening self-esteem. Service models in which a person has an opportunity to help others as well as being helped might be successful. Support groups (popular with younger women with breast cancer) may not appeal to many women in later adulthood.

The experience of breast cancer presents a woman with several "tasks" that are quite similar to the developmental tasks of persons in later adulthood. Self-absorption, depression, dealing with an uncertain future, and learning to balance hope and despair are tasks faced by women with breast cancer and by the elderly. For those women who have already worked through the issue of reviewing and accepting one's life and developing a viewpoint about death and avoiding depression, breast cancer may not be so difficult to "take in one's stride." Women who have not had life-threatening experiences earlier in the life course or who are socially isolated, however, may experience a more difficult adjustment with an extended period of self-absorption and depression.

In the introduction to this book, we mentioned that older women were underrepresented in our study sample. The reasons for this underrepresentation may relate to some of the themes discussed in this chapter. Because we sought subjects through organizations that serve breast cancer patients, we may have failed to locate those older women whose strong sense of independence keeps them from participating in the activities of these organizations. Women who want to minimize the problem, and face it with a stiff upper lip, were not likely to hear our call for volunteers. Those suffering depression, those whose past experiences allowed them to take breast cancer in their stride, and those with other more debilitating illness were probably less likely to be attending the programs where we sought volunteers.

It is also possible that physicians and other health providers are less likely to refer their older patients to these programs. They may assume they [older women] do not need help or simply take the problems of these women less seriously. As breast cancer has been equated in the public mind with the loss of a breast, and not so much with the underlying disease, health practitioners may erroneously conclude that older women have an easy time adjusting to breast cancer. As we have shown in this chapter, this is not necessarily the case. Older women are still sexual beings, and their self-image can be seriously affected by mastectomy. Some older women will be subject to depression and anxiety. Many older women do not have the social support resources of younger women. Organizations that serve breast cancer patients may need to examine their services in light of the needs of their older patients and assure that services are available that meet the needs of this population.

7 Conclusion

One of our goals, in writing this book, was to allow women to share their experiences with breast cancer and its treatment. Even though breast cancer is widespread, we live in a society where the words "cancer" and "breast" remain to some extent unmentionable. As a result, women have been prevented from gaining access to the experiences of other women—the raw material women most need to learn. By focusing on breast cancer *as it is experienced by women*, we have also learned some lessons that we believe could help health professionals, and, before going on to discuss our major conclusions, we would like to review several of these.

By listening to the voices of women with breast cancer, we have learned that some areas of importance to women have been underemphasized. For example, in medical care, more attention has been given to the breast as an object of sexual desire than to it as a source of sexual pleasure. Women in our sample were concerned about the loss of an erogenous zone, something that is not restored by reconstruction. Recently, doctors have learned to remove the prostate surgically without cutting the nerves to the penis, thereby preserving sexuality in men with prostate cancer. Could doctors work on developing a mastectomy that would preserve feeling in the breast area?

Women were also concerned about the effect of the cancer and its treatments on their fertility. Even women who had completed their families were grieved by the loss of fertility brought on by chemotherapy and hormone treatments. These treatments also interfered with sexuality, decreasing libido and vaginal secretions. Most women in our sample were unprepared for these changes and had no help in dealing with them. Clearly, more attention needs to be paid to the areas of fertility and sexuality.

Another disparity we observed by listening to women is that most professional literature on breast cancer focuses on the *psychological* impact, whereas women focus more heavily on the *social* aspects. Women place a high value on relationships with others, often putting the needs of others above their own. Social relationships are also a major contributor to successful adaptation to breast cancer. Service providers for breast cancer patients need to explore how this powerful resource can be used to benefit women. For example, many women panicked at some point during radiation treatments (a lonely experience), whereas others received support from a chemotherapy program that was set up like a beauty parlor which facilited connectedness. More attention needs to be given to building social relationships into the treatment of breast cancer. Because women tend to think first of others, women of all ages with breast cancer need encouragement to ask more directly for what they need *from others* (husbands, partners, friends, mothers, and children) to help them cope with this crisis.

It is also clear, from listening to women with breast cancer, that there is no single solution or "best way" to handle all women. With respect to current controversies about treatment choices, there is no single choice or way of making that choice that is right for every woman. Some women *do* want their physicians to make the decision for them, but many do not. Some want lots of time to process the information, and some just want to get the procedure done. Some place high value on appearance and may want reconstruction done simultaneously with the mastectomy. Others care more about the impact on their fertility or their life goals and plans. Some want to be surrounded by cheerful, optimistic people, and others want to be allowed to grieve. Many will want different things at different times. When Freud asked, "What do women want?" he was asking the same question many health providers ask today. This is not the right question, however. Women need to be understood as individuals, with unique styles and situations. Each woman should be asked what *she* wants, and above all, she must be listened to.

Before moving on to the conclusions regarding our main thesis, we want to point out that at every life stage, the breast cancer experience provided women with both challenges and opportunities for personal growth. In general, the breast cancer tasks become more compatible with the life-course tasks as women get older. In the 20s and 30s, the requirements for successful adaptation to breast cancer can conflict with life-development tasks. For example, the young woman's need to commit herself to intimate relationships, children, and careers can be made more difficult when breast cancer pushes her to self-absorption, dependency, and knowledge of an uncertain future. In midlife and later adulthood, the tasks of life development and breast cancer are more similar. This is not to say that adaptation is necessarily easier for older women, because when these forces hit simultaneously, they may be overwhelming and more difficult to overcome. It does seem, however, that adaptation to breast cancer is easiest for a woman who has *already* successfully resolved the tasks brought on by the illness. A woman who has already given up the idea of a just world and who has developed a viewpoint about death is less likely to experience anger and depression than one for whom these are new tasks. Although this can be a woman of any age, it is most likely to be an older woman.

In writing this book, we wanted to explore the question of whether breast cancer is experienced differently by women of different ages. Our goal was not to determine whether adjustment to breast cancer was easier for younger women or for older women, but rather to discover whether different aspects of the experience were more salient to women at different places in the life course. What emerged can best be described with an analogy to a perennial garden. All of the plants are in the garden throughout the growing season, but different plants come into flower at different times. Observing the garden at different points in the season, one sees all of the plants, but one's attention is drawn to the plants in flower at the time. We can think of the plants as the tasks of serious illness. All of the tasks are there for every woman with breast cancer, regardless of age. Each woman must manage the psychological reactions of anxiety, depression, and self-absorption. Each must try to find a balance between hope and despair. All must learn to preserve a satisfactory body image, maintain satisfactory sexual relationships, adjust to role shifts, and deal with an uncertain future. In different life stages, however, different tasks come into sharper focus and seem to occupy more of the attention of the women in this stage.

Women who are diagnosed with breast cancer in their 20s are striving for autonomy from their families of origin. When the illness requires more dependency, role shifts that involve greater reliance on the family of origin are common. The young woman may be very troubled by this, seeing any dependence as a kind of failure. For the young woman who has not yet had children, breast cancer may bring the issue of her fertility to the forefront, and some change in life goals may be needed concerning children. The task of managing the psychological reaction of self-absorption, which is common in any illness, is especially important to the young woman with breast cancer, because too much self-absorption can interfere with the achievement of intimacy, an important life task in this life stage. Finally, young women with breast cancer may find that the task of dealing with an uncertain future intersects with a need to find a place in the adult world. In some cases, breast cancer may make the achievement of a dream impossible. In other cases, heightened awareness that the future is uncertain may spur a young woman on toward fulfilling a dream that had been earlier postponed.

For women in their 30s, a different set of tasks emerges. The psychological reaction that looms large at this age is anger, which stems from the intersection of believing that the world is fair and getting breast cancer. Women with breast cancer in their 30s need to learn to let go of the idea that the world is just and accompanying anger. Another psychological reaction of importance to women in their 30s who have young children is self-absorption. Self-absorption can interfere with the ability to nurture young children. The task of dealing with an uncertain future can make it difficult for a young mother with breast cancer to provide her children with a sense of security and trust. Because sexuality is often at a peak for women in their 30s, the task of maintaining satisfactory sexual relationships is especially important at this life stage. Women in their 30s can also experience difficulties in relationships with their mothers. Although the illness may create increased dependency needs in the young adult woman, by the 30s, she seems to have created a degree of independence that precludes a return to a "pretransitional" relationship with her mother where the daughter is more dependent. Women in their 30s tend to both wish for more nurturing from their mothers and at the same time to reject nurturance that is offered. Nor do these women, as a whole, have strong support from husbands, partners, or friends. Thus, they have little help in adapting to any role shifts necessitated by the illness. Like women in their 20s, life goals for women in their 30s were affected by the need to deal with an uncertain future. Many women in the 30s are already reassessing their roles, shifting from a focus on family to work, or vice versa. For some women in their 30s, breast cancer seems to offer a legitimate reason to move off the career fast track and focus on relationships and families. Cancer may help these women to have confidence in their own values rather than accepting the values of the dominant culture, which emphasizes career accomplishment over relationships.

For midlife women, who are already dealing with an aging body, the breast cancer task of preserving a satisfactory body image takes on special importance. Marriages are also under severe strain in midlife, and breast cancer puts additional pressures on the marriage because of the need to adapt to role shifts. Because of the wife's need for emotional support at this time, traditional marriages, in which husbands perform instrumental roles, are especially vulnerable. Another intersection of life tasks and illness tasks in midlife occurs in the area of parenting adolescent children. At this point in their lives, children need to separate from the family of origin, and parents need to let go and help their children to achieve autonomy. Women with breast cancer may want to lean on their adolescent children for emotional support, however, breast cancer seems to make the transition to independence particularly difficult for adolescent daughters. A midlife woman may also seek social support from her mother or from her friends. Because women have so often been providers of social support rather than recipients, many have difficulty asking for this support and often feel hurt when it does not materialize. As a result of their experience with breast cancer, some midlife women move to a new level of self-reliance and learn to better assure that their own needs are being met.

The midlife tasks of confronting death, reassessment and generativity also intersect with breast cancer tasks (Table 7.1). While midlife women are confronting their mortality, breast cancer patients must learn to deal with an uncertain future. These tasks are very similar, and the result can be an overemphasis on mortality, leading to depression, or a constructive

Table 7.1 Themes of Women with Breast Cancer in Young, Middle, and Later Adulthood

---

Young Adulthood (Phase 1): The Twenties

    Achieving independence
    Fertility
    Developing intimate relationships
    Establishing a place in the adult world

Young Adulthood (Phase 2): The Thirties
    Letting go of the just world idea
    Sexuality
    Coping with children
    Relationships with mothers
    Evaluating the meaning of work

Midlife
    Body image
    Marriage
    Relationships with adolescent children
    Confronting death
    Reassessing one's life
    Self-reliance
    Generativity
    Relationships with mothers
    Friendships

Late Adulthood
    Coping with loss
    Relationships with children
    Independence
    Depression-despair

---

acceptance of mortality, leading to personal growth. Along the same vein, the midlife task of "reassessment" is very similar to the process in which breast cancer patients find new meaning in life. The self-absorption that is common in serious illness can facilitate the resolution of this task. Generativity is viewed as the positive resolution to the psychosocial crisis of midlife (Erikson, 1980), and breast cancer can provide a context in which this resolution can occur. Many midlife women in our sample are the backbone of local volunteer programs for breast cancer patients. In some cases, however, self-absorption can make generativity difficult to achieve.

In later adulthood, many women are coping with losses, such as loss of spouse, job, and health. Breast cancer poses a similar task, necessitating adaptation to loss of good health and, for many women, loss of a breast. In cases in which a woman has had an overwhelming series of losses, or has not yet developed good coping mechanisms for handling loss, this may be especially difficult. In later adulthood, a woman may become increasingly dependent on her children, especially when illness strikes. Breast cancer can also require role shifts involving increased dependency. It is important that older women receive the help and support they need without losing any more independence than necessary, as maintaining independence is very important to the self-esteem of the elderly. In life development theory, older adults go through a process of life review and develop a viewpoint about death. They can reach a level of satisfaction and integrity, or they can experience despair. In breast cancer in later adulthood, the process of life review can be facilitated by self-absorption, but depression may make it very difficult for the older woman to avoid despair.

Several illness tasks are particularly important in one life stage (e.g., sexuality in the 30s, body image in midlife), whereas others seem to run through the life course, important in different ways at different life stages. One of the latter is role shifts, highlighting the issue of independence. Young women (20s) strive for independence, and older women (60+) struggle to maintain it. For women in their 30s, preserving independence can mean a denial of dependency needs. In midlife, women seem to be more comfortable accepting their dependency and often reach out for support, but at this point in life, support may not be available. Women of all ages need to learn to build support networks for themselves (as the lesbian women in our sample had done), because the traditional family does not always do a good job of providing socioemotional support for women.

We found evidence of conflict between mothers and daughters throughout the life course, with breast cancer serving to complicate this already highly complex relationship further. Mothers who tried to nurture adult daughters with breast cancer were often rejected. If they were not supportive, however, daughters felt let down. When daughters tried to support mothers with breast cancer, mothers often felt the daughters were trying to take control. In many cases, a kind of power struggle seemed to be going on, with both parties wanting both nurturance, and indepencence or control. Although breast cancer did not create these conflicts, it heightened women's need for support and at the same time prevented them from being able to provide support. Guilt concerning the possible genetic nature of the disease often made direct communication between mothers and daughters even more difficult.

Another issue that was important to breast cancer patients throughout the life course was the need to deal with an uncertain future. Virtually every woman we interviewed went through a process of reassessment in which basic values were reaffirmed and priorities were clarified. Women came to feel that if their life might be limited, they would learn to live every moment to the fullest. For some women, this meant doing something *now* that they had thought they would get to at some unspecified time in the future. For others, it meant letting go of goals they had been pursuing and enjoying life more. For most, it meant giving more time to important relationships and to meeting their own needs. For some, it meant letting go of goals altogether and learning to live fully in the moment.

In sharing their feelings, the women we interviewed provide models not only for other women with breast cancer but for all of us. Breast cancer serves as a startling reminder of what is, after all, the human condition. We are all dying. We *all* live with an uncertain future. The woman with breast cancer is shaken out of the waking dream the rest of us live in and forced to come to grips with a future we all share. The sheer courage with which these women rise to the task is inspiring. Although courage is something that is traditionally thought of as a male virtue, and associated with guns and war, these women face their illness and its terrifying treatments, surviving panic and depression, to emerge with a philosophy that allows them to get up every morning, go through the routine motions of daily living, provide loving care for their husbands, children, partners, families, and friends, all the while knowing that their cancer could recur at any time. Because they are aware that life is not guaranteed, it becomes more precious to them, and in this way, they provide a model for living fully from which we all can learn.

REFERENCES

Adams, D. (1984). The psychosocial development of professional black women's lives and the consequences of career for their personal happiness. (Doctoral dissertation, Wright Institute, Berkeley, CA, 1983). *Dissertation Abstracts International, 44,* 12.

Ainlay, S. C., & Smith, R. (1984). Aging and religious participation. *Journal of Gerontology, 39,* 357–363.

Alagaratnam, T. T., & Kung, N. Y. (1986). Psychosocial effects of mastectomy: Is it due to mastectomy or to the diagnosis of malignancy? *British Journal of Psychiatry, 149,* 296–299.

American Cancer Society. (1990). *Cancer facts and figures—1989.* Atlanta, GA: Author.

Ariel, I. M., & Cleary, J. B. (1986). *Breast cancer diagnosis and treatment.* New York: McGraw Hill.

Asken, M. (1975). Psychoemotional aspects of mastectomy: A review of recent literature. *American Journal of Psychiatry, 132,* 56–59.

Atchley, R. C. (1980). *The social forces in later life.* Belmont, CA: Wadsworth.

Baider, L., Rizel, S., & DeNour, A. K. (1986). Comparison of couples' adjustment to lumpectomy and mastectomy. *General Hospital Psychiatry, 8,* 251–257.

Bankoff, E. (1978, November). *Support from family and friends: What helps the widow.* Paper presented at the Thirty-second Annual Scientific Meeting of the Gerontological Society, Washington, DC.

Bankoff, E. (1983). Aged parents and their widowed daughters: A support relationship. *Journal of Gerontology, 38,* 226–230.

Bard, M., & Sutherland, A. M. (1955). Psychological impact of cancer and its treatment: 4. Adaptation to radical mastectomy. *Cancer, 8,* 652–672.

Bartelink, H., Van Dam, F., & VanDongen, J. (1985). Psychological effects of breast conserving therapy in comparison with radical mastectomy. *International Journal of Radiation Oncology, Biology, Physics, 11,* 381–385.

Baruch, G., Barnett, R., & Rivers, C. (1983). *Life prints: New patterns of love and work for today's woman.* New York: McGraw-Hill.

Baumann, L. A. (1988). Adolescents' perception of and adaptation to mother's breast cancer. *Oncology Nursing Forum, 15* (Suppl. 2), 129.

Beck, C. M., & Pearson, B. P. (1989). Mental health of elderly women. *Journal of Women and Aging, 1,* (1, 2, 3) 175–193.

Beckmann, J., Johansen, L., & Blichert-Teft, M. (1983). Psychological reactions in younger women operated on for breast cancer: Amputation versus resection of the breast with special reference to body image, sexual identity and sexual function. *Danish Medical Bulletin, 30*(2), 10–13.

Belenky, M. P., Clinchy, B. M., Goldberger, N. R., Tarule, J. M. (1986). *Women's ways of knowing: The development of self, voice and mind.* New York: Basic Books.

Berger, J. (1984). Crisis intervention: A drop-in support group for cancer patients and their families. *Social Work in Health Care, 10*(2), 81–92.

Bergholz, E. (1988, December). Under the shadow of cancer. *The New York Times Magazine,* pp. 73–85.

Blazyk, S., & Canavan, M. M. (1986). Managing the discharge crisis following catastrophic illness or injury. *Social Work in Health Care, 11*(4), 19–32.

Block, M., Davidson, J., & Grambs, J. (1981). *Women over forty: Visions and realities.* New York: Springer Publishing Co.

Bloom, J. R. (1982). Social support, accommodation to stress and adjustment to breast cancer. *Social Science and Medicine, 16,* 1329–1338.

Bloom, J. R., Cook, M., Fotopoulos, S., Flamer, D., Gates, C., Holland, J. C., Muenz, L., Murawski, B., Penman, D., & Ross, R. D. (1987). Psychological response to mastectomy: A prospective comparison study. *Cancer, 59,* 189–196.

Bloom, J. R., & Spiegel, D. (1984). The relationship of two dimensions of social support to the psychological well being and social functioning of women with advanced breast cancer. *Social Science and Medicine, 19*(8), 831–837.

Blumberg, B., Flaherty, M., & Lewis, J. (Eds.). (1982). *Coping with cancer: A resource for the health professional* (NIH Publication No. 82-2080). Bethesda, MD: National Cancer Institute.

Boston Women's Health Book Collective. (1973). *Our bodies, ourselves.* Boston: Simon and Schuster.

Boudreau, J. A. (1988). Women with mastectomies and reconstructive surgery: Body satisfaction self-esteem, depression, life satisfaction and outlook. *Dissertation Abstracts International,* [B]; *49*(2), 537. Order # AAD88-06503.

Brady, M. L. (1987). Psychological interactions for women with breast disease. *Obstetrics and Gynecology Clinics of North America, 14,* 797–816.

Bransfield, D. D. (1982). Breast cancer and sexual functioning: A review of the literature and implications for future research. *International Journal of Psychiatry in Medicine, 12,* 197–211.

Brody, E. (1981). Women in the middle and family help to older people. *The Gerontologist, 21,* 471–480.

Brody, E. (1985). Parent care as a normative stress. *The Gerontologist, 25,* 19–29.

Brody, E., Johnson, P., & Fulcomer, M. (1984). What should adult children do for elderly parents? Opinions and preferences of three generations of women. *Journal of Gerontology, 39,* 736–746.

Brown, P. L. (1987, Sept. 14). Studying seasons of a woman's life. *The New York Times,* B17.

Buckley, I. G. (1979). *Listen to the children: A study of the impact on the mental health of children of a parent's catastrophic illness.* New York: Cancer Care.

Bumagin, V., & Hirn, K. (1982). Observations on changing relationships for older married women. *American Journal of Psychoanalysis, 42,* 140–146.

Burgess, C., Morris, T., & Pettingale, K. W. (1988). Psychological response to cancer diagnosis: II. Evidence for coping styles. *Journal of Psychosomatic Research, 32,* 263–272.

Burish, T., & Lyles, J. N. (1983). Coping with the effects of cancer treatments. In T. G. Burish & L. A. Bradley (Eds.), *Coping with chronic disease: Research and applications* (pp. 161–189). New York: Academic Press.

Burkhalter, P. K. (1978). Sexuality and the cancer patient. In P. K. Burkhalter & D. L. Donely (Eds.), *Dynamics of oncology nursing* (pp. 249–274). New York: McGraw-Hill.

Byrd, B. F. (1975). Sex after mastectomy. *Medical Aspects of Human Sexuality, 9*, 53–54.

Campbell, S. (1984). The fifty-year-old woman and midlife stress. *International Journal of Aging and Human Development, 18*, 295–307.

Cantor, M. (1983). Strain among caregivers: A study of experiences in the United States. *The Gerontologist, 23*, 597–604.

Carroll, R. M. (1981). The impact of mastectomy on body image. *Oncology Nursing Forum, 8*, 29–32.

Carter, E., & McGoldrick, M. (1980). *The family life cycle: A framework for family therapy.* New York: Gardner.

Carter, E., & McGoldrick, M. (Eds.). (1989). *The changing family life cycle: A framework for family therapy.* New York: Gardner.

Chodorow, N. (1978). *The reproduction of mothering: Psychoanalysis and the sociology of gender.* Berkeley: University of California.

Clifford, E. (1979). The reconstruction experience: The search for restitution. In N. G. Georgrade (Ed.), *Breast reconstruction following mastectomy* (pp. 22–34). St. Louis: C. V. Mosby.

Cobb, S. (1976). Social support as a moderator of life stress. *Psychosomatic Medicine, 38*, 300–314.

Cohen, S., & Syme, S. L. (1985). *Social support and health.* New York: Academic Press.

Colarusso, C. A., & Nemiroff, R. A. (1981). *Adult development.* New York: Plenum.

Cooper, C. L., Cooper, R., & Faragher, E. B. (1989). Incidence and perception of psychosocial stress: The relationship with breast cancer. *Psychological Medicine, 19*, 415–422.

Cox, E. (1984). Breast Cancer: 1. Practice: Psychological aspects. *Nursing Mirror, 159*, 18–19.

Craig, T. J., & Abecoff, M. D. (1974). Psychiatric symptomotology among hospitalized cancer patients. *American Journal of Psychiatry, 131*, 1323–1327.

Craig, T. J., Comstock, G. W., & Geiser, P. B. (1974). The quality of survival in breast cancer: A case control comparison. *Cancer, 33*, 1451–1457.

Cumming, E., & Henry, W. E. (1961). *Growing old.* New York: Basic Books.

Davis, K. (1978). Mastectomy: Treating the total woman. *Sexual Medicine Today, 2*, 38–47.

Deadman, J. M., Dewey, M. J., Owens, R. G., Leinster, S. J., & Slade, P. D. (1989). Threat and loss in breast cancer. *Psychological Medicine, 19*, 677–681.

Dean, C. (1988). The emotional impact of mastectomy. *British Journal of Hospital Medicine, 39*, 30–32, 36, 38–39.

Dean, C., & Surtees, P. G. (1989). Do psychological factors predict survival in breast cancer? *Journal of Psychosomatic Research, 33*, 561–569.

Derogatis, L. R., & Kowalesis, S. M. (1981). An approach to evaluation of sexual problems in the cancer patient. *Cancer—A Cancer Journal for Clinicians, 31*, 46–50.

Easley, E. B. (1983). Important facts about the menopause. *North Carolina Medical Journal, 44*, 369–375.

Erikson, E. (1978). *Adulthood.* New York: Norton.

Erikson, E. (1980). *Identity and the life cycle* (rev. ed.). New York: Norton.

Erikson, E. (1982). *The life cycle completed: A review.* New York: Norton.

Euster, S. (1979). Rehabilitation after mastectomy: The group process. *Social Work in Health Care, 4,* 251–263.

Fallowfield, L. J., Baum, M., & Maguire, G. P. (1986). Effects of breast conservation on psychological morbidity associated with diagnosis and treatment of early breast cancer. *British Medical Journal, 293,* 1331–1334.

Feather, B. L., & Wainstock, J. M. (1989a). Perceptions of postmastectomy patients: 1. The relationships between social support and network providers. *Cancer Nursing, 12,* 293–300.

Feather, B. L., & Wainstock, J. M. (1989b). Perceptions of postmastectomy patients: 2. Social support and attitudes toward mastectomy. *Cancer Nursing, 12,* 301–309.

Fidell, L. (1980). Sex role stereotypes and the American physician. *Psychology of Women Quarterly, 4,* 313–330.

Finch, D. P., & Marshall, J. (1983). The role of stress, social support and age in survival from breast cancer. *Journal of Psychosomatic Research, 27,* 77–83.

Finlayson, A. (1976). Social networks as coping resources. *Social Science and Medicine, 10,* 97–103.

Fischer, L. R. (1986). *Linked lives: Adult daughters and their mothers.* New York: Harper & Row.

Fisher, B. (1985). Choice of surgery in early breast cancer. *Conference on early breast cancer: The psychological perspective.* New York: Long Island Jewish Medical Center and Memorial Sloan-Kettering Cancer Center.

Fisher, B., & Barboni, P. (1982). Breast cancer. In J. F. Holland & E. Frei III (Eds.), *Cancer medicine* (pp. 2025–2056). Philadelphia: Lea & Febiger.

Fisher, B., Redmond, C., Fisher, E. R., Banoz, M., Wolmark, N., Wickerham, D. L., Deutsch, M., Montague, E., Margolese, R., & Foster, R. (1985). Ten-year results of a randomized clinical trial comparing radical mastectomy and total mastectomy with or without radiation. *New England Journal of Medicine, 312,* 674–681.

Fisher, B., Redmond, C., Poisson, R., Margolese, R., Wolmark, N., Wickerham, L., Fisher, E., Deutsch, M., Caplan, R., Pilch, Y., Slass, A., Shibata, H., Lerner, H., Terz, J., & Sidorovich, L. (1989). Eight-year results of a randomized clinical trial comparing total mastectomy and lumpectomy with or without irradiation in the treatment of breast cancer. *New England Journal of Medicine, 320*(13), 822–28.

Fisher, B., Redmond, C., Wolmark, N., & Wieand, H. S. (1981). Disease-free survival at intervals during and following completion of adjuvant chemotherapy: The NSABP experience from three breast cancer protocol. *Cancer, 48,* 1273–1280.

Fisher, B., Slack, N., Katrych, D., & Wolmark, N. (1975). Ten-year follow-up results of patients with carcinoma of the breast in a co-operative clinical trial evaluating surgical adjuvant chemotherapy. *Surgery, Gynecology and Obstetrics, 140,* 528–534.

Flynn, K. T., & Shannon, R. M. (1987). Survivors of cancer: Finding meaning in illness. *Oncology Nursing Forum, 14,* 153.

Folkman, S., Lazarus, R. S., Pimley, S., & Novacek, J. (1987). Age differences in stress and coping processes. *Psychology and Aging, 2,* 171–184.

Fox, B. H. (1983). Current theory of psychogenic effects on cancer incidence and prognosis. *Journal of Psychosocial Oncology, 1*(1), 17.

Freeman, E. L., Cash, T., & Wirstead, B. (1984). *Perceived changes in physical self-concept and marital and sexual relations in patients who have had mastectomy and breast reconstruction surgery.* Paper presented at the annual meeting of the Society of Behavioral Medicine, Philadelphia, May.

Friedman, L. C., Baer, P. E., Nelson, D. V., Lane, M., Smith, F. E., & Dworkin, R. J. (1988). Women with breast cancer: Perception of family functioning and adjustment to illness. *Psychomatic Medicine, 50,* 529–540.

Garner, J. D., & Mercer, S. O. (Eds.). (1989). *Women as they age: Challenge, opportunity, and triumph.* Binghamton, NY: Haworth.

Gates, C. C. (1988). The "most-significant-other" in the care of the breast cancer patient. *Cancer, 38,* 146–153.

Gerard, D. (1982). Sexual functioning after mastectomy: Life vs. lab. *Journal of Sex and Marital Therapy, 8,* 305–315.

Giacquinta, B. (1977). Helping families face the crisis of cancer. *American Journal of Nursing, 77,* 1585–1588.

Giele, J. (Ed.). (1982). *Women in the middle years.* New York: Wiley.

Gilligan, C. (1982a). Adult development and women's development: Arrangements for a marriage. In J. Giele (Ed.), *Women in the middle years* (pp. 89–114). New York: Wiley.

Gilligan, C. (1982b). *In a different voice.* Cambridge, MA: Harvard University.

Glasser, B. G., & Strauss, A. L. (1967). *The discovery of grounded theory.* Chicago: Aldine.

Goin, M. K., & Goin, J. M. (1981). Midlife reactions to mastectomy and subsequent breast reconstruction. *Archives of General Psychiatry, 38,* 25–227.

Golan, N. (1981). *Passing through transitions.* New York: Free Press.

Goleman, D. (1990, February 6). Compassion and comfort in middle age. *The New York Times,* pp. C1, C14.

Goldberg, R. J., & Tull, R. M. (1983). *The psychosocial dimensions of cancer.* New York: Free Press.

Gordon, W. A., Freidenberger, I., Diller, L., Hibbard, M., Wolf, L., Levise, L., Lipkins, R., Ezrachi, O. J., & Lucidi, D. (1980). Efficacy of psychosocial intervention with cancer patients. *Journal of Consulting and Clinical Psychology, 48,* 743–759.

Gotay, C. C. (1984). The experience of cancer during early and advanced stages: The views of patients and their mates. *Social Science and Medicine, 18,* 605–613.

Gotay, C. C. (1985). Why me? Attributions and adjustment by cancer patients and their families at two stages in the disease process. *Social Science and Medicine, 20,* 825–831.

Gould, R. L. (1978). *Transformations: Growth and change in adult life.* New York: Simon and Schuster.

Graham, J. (1982). *In the company of others.* New York: Harcourt Brace Jovanovich.

Grandstaff, N. W. (1976). The impact of breast cancer on the family. *Frontiers of Radiation Therapy and Oncology, 11,* 145–156.

Graydon, J. E. (1984). Breast cancer: Stress points. *American Journal of Nursing, 84*, 1124.

Greer, S., & Morris, T. (1978). The study of psychological factors in breast cancer. *Social Science and Medicine, 12*, 129–174.

Griffith, J. W. (1983). Women's stress responses and coping patterns according to age groups. 2. *Issues in Health Care of Women, 6*, 327–340.

Grossarth-Maticek, R., & Eysenck, H. J. (1989). Length of survival and lymphocyte percentage in women with mammary cancer as a function of psychotherapy. *Psychological Reports, 65*, 315–321.

Gyelensköld, K. (1982). *Breast cancer: The psychological effects of the disease and its treatment.* New York: Methuen.

Hailey, B. J., Lavine, B., & Hogan, B. (1988). The mastectomy experience: Patients' perspectives. *Women and Health, 14*(1), 75–88.

Heim, E., Augustiny, K. F., Blaser, A., Burki, C., Kuhne, D., Rothenbuhler, M., Schaffner, L., & Valach, L. (1987). Coping with breast cancer: A longitudinal prospective study. *Psychotherapy and Psychosomatics, 48*, 44–59.

Holland, J. C. (1973) Psychologic aspects of cancer. In J. C. Holland & E. Frei III (Eds.), *Cancer medicine* (pp. 991–1021). Philadelphia: Lea & Febiger.

Holland, J. C. (1984). The psychological and social effects of cancer. In L. Roberts (Ed.), *Cancer today: Origins, prevention, and treatment* (pp. 91–101). Washington, DC: Institute of Medicine.

Holland, J. C. (1976). Coping with cancer: A challenge to the behavioral sciences. In J. W. Cullen, B. H. Fox, & R. N. Isom (Eds.), *Cancer: The behavioral dimensions* (pp. 1–3, 7) (DHEW Publication No. [NIH] 76–1074). Bethesda, MD: National Cancer Institute.

Holland, J. C. (1977). Psychological management of cancer patients and their families. *Practical Psychology*, 14–20.

Holland, J. C., & Mastrovito, R. (1980). Psychological adaptation to breast cancer. *Cancer, 46*, 1045–1052.

Holland, J. C. & Rowland, J. H. (1987). Psychological reactions to breast cancer and its treatment. In J. R. Harris, S. Hellman, I. C. Henderson, & D. W. Kinne (Eds.), *Breast diseases* (pp. 632–647). Philadelphia: Lippincott.

Holland, J. C., Rowland, J. H., Lebovits, A., & Rusalem, R. (1979). Reactions to cancer treatment: Assessment of emotional response to adjuvant radiotherapy as a guide to planned interventions. *Psychiatric Clinics of North America, 2*, 347–358.

Holmberg, L., Omne-Ponten, M., Burns, T., Adami, H. O., & Bergstrom, R. (1989). Psychosocial adjustment after mastectomy and breast-conserving treatment. *Cancer, 64*, 969–974.

Holzer, C. E., Leaf, P. J., & Weissman, M. M. (1985). Living with depression. In M. R. Haug, A. B. Ford, & M. Sheafer (Eds.), *The psychological and mental health of aged women* (pp. 101–116). New York: Springer.

Hubbs-Tait, L. (1989). Coping patterns of aging women: A developmental perspective. In J. Garner & S. Mercer (Eds.), *Women as they age* (pp. 95–121). New York: Haworth.

Hughson, A. V., Cooper, A. F., McArdle, C. S., & Smith, D. C. (1987). Psychosocial effects of radiotherapy after mastectomy. *British Medical Journal, 294*(6586), 1515–1518.

Hughson, A. V., Cooper, A. F., McArdle, C. S., & Smith, D. C. (1988). Psychosocial morbidity in patients awaiting breast biopsy. *Journal of Psychosomatic Research, 32,* 173–180.

Jamison, R. N., Burish, T. G., & Wallston, K. A. (1987). Psychogenic factors in predicting survival of breast cancer patients. *Journal of Clinical Oncology, 5,* 768–772.

Jamison, K., Wellisch, D. K., & Pasnau, R. D. (1978). Psychosocial aspects of mastectomy: The woman's perspective. *American Journal of Psychiatry, 135,* 432–436.

Jenks, J. (1983). The mystery of women's early development. *Clinical Social Work Journal, 11,* 52–63.

Jensen, M. R. (1987). Psychobiological factors predicting the course of breast cancer. *Journal of Personality, 55,* 317–342.

Johnson, C., & Connors, M. (1987). *The etiology and treatment of bulimia nervosa.* New York: Basic Books.

Johnson, J. (1987). *Intimacy: Living as a woman after cancer.* Toronto, Canada: N C Press Limited.

Jung, C. (1933). *Modern man in search of a soul.* New York: Harcourt, Brace.

Kaas, M. J. (1987). *Emotional referencing: The definition and management of mental health by older women* (University Microfilms). San Francisco: University of California (ADG 87-23874).

Kahana, B., & Kahana, E. (1982). Clinical issues of middle age and later life. *The Annals of the American Academy of Political and Social Science, 464,* 140–161.

Kalish, R. A. (1976). Death and dying in a social context. In R. H. Binstock & E. Shanas (Eds.), *Handbook of aging and the social sciences* (pp. 149–170). New York: Van Nostrand Reinhold.

Karp, D. A. (1988). A decade of reminders: Changing age consciousness between fifty and sixty years old. *The Gerontologist, 28,* 727–738.

Kasl, S. V., & Berkman, L. S. (1981). Some psycho-social influences on the health status of the elderly: The perspective of social epidemiology. In J. L. McGaugh and S. B. Kiesler (Eds.), *Aging: Biology and behavior* (pp. 345–385). New York: Academic Press.

Katz, J. L., Weiner, H., Gallagher, T. F., & Hellman, L. (1970). Stress, distress, and ego defenses. *Archives of General Psychiatry, 23,* 131–142.

Kemeny, M. M., Wellisch, D. K., & Schain, W. S. (1988). Psychosocial outcome in a randomized surgical trial for treatment of primary breast cancer. *Cancer, 62,* 1231–1237.

Kerber, A. K. (1987). Locus of control, hope, and disease-free interval. *Oncology Nursing Forum, 14*(2), 121.

Klagsbrun, S. C. (1970). Cancer, emotions, and nurses. *American Journal of Psychiatry, 126,* 1237–1244.

Krouse, H. J., & Krouse, J. H. (1982). Cancer as crisis: The critical elements of adjustment. *Nursing Research, 31,* 96–101.

Kulys, R., & Tobin, S. S. (1980). Interpreting the lack of future planning among the elderly. *International Journal of Aging and Human Development. 11*(2), 111–126.

Kushner, R. (1975). *Breast cancer: A personal history and investigative report.* New York: Harcourt Brace Jovanovich.

Leiber, L., Plumb, M. M., Gestenzang, M. L. & Holland, J. (1976). The communication of affection between cancer patients and their spouses. *Psychosomatic Medicine, 38,* 379–389.

Lerner, H. G. (1985). *The dance of anger.* New York: Harper & Row.

Levinson, D. J., Darrow, C. N., Klein, E., Levinson, M., & McKee, B. (1978). *The seasons of a man's life.* New York: Random House.

Levy, S. M., Herberman, R. B., Lee, J. K., Lippman, M. E., & d'Angelo, T. (1989). Breast conservation versus mastectomy: Distress sequelae as a function of choice. *Journal of Clinical Oncology, 7,* 367–375.

Levy, S. M., Herberman, R. B., Whiteside, T., Sanzo, K., Lee, J., & Kirwood, J. (1990). Perceived social support and tumor estrogen/progesterone receptor status as predictors of natural killer cell activity in breast cancer cell patients. *Psychosomatic Medicine, 52,* 73–85.

Levy, S. M., Herberman, R., & Winkelstein, A. (1987). Natural killer cell activity in primary breast cancer patients: Social and behavioral predictors. Presented at the Annual Meeting of the American *Society of Clinical Oncology, 6,* A1019.

Lewis, F. M., Ellison, E. S., & Woods, N. F. (1985). The impact of breast cancer on the family. *Seminars in Oncology Nursing, 1,* 206–213.

Lichtman, R. R., Taylor, S. E., Wood, J. V., Bluming, A. Z., Dosik, G. M., & Liebowitz, R. L. (1984). Relations with children after breast cancer. The mother-daughter relationship at risk. *Journal of Psychosocial Oncology, 2*(3, 4), 1–19.

Lidz, T. (1980). Phases of adult life: an overview. In W. Norman & T. Scaramella (Eds.), *Mid-life: Developmental and clinical issues* (pp. 20–37). New York: Brunner-Mazel.

Lifshitz, L. H. (Ed.). (1988). *Women's poetry on breast cancer: Her soul beneath the bone.* Chicago: University of Illinois.

Lifton, R. J. (1979). *The broken connection.* New York: Simon and Schuster.

Lindsey, A. M., Norbeck, J. S., Carrieri, V. L., & Perry, E. (1981). Social support and health outcomes in postmastectomy women: A review. *Cancer Nursing, 4,* 377–384.

Litman, T. J. (1974). The family as the basic unit in health and medical care: A social behavioral overview. *Social Science and Medicine, 8,* 495.

Litwak, E. (1981). *The modified extended family, social networks, and research continuities in aging.* New York: Center for Sciences at Columbia University.

Love, R. R., Leventhal, H., Easterling, D. V., & Nerenz, D. R. (1989). Side effects and emotional distress during cancer chemotherapy. *Cancer, 63,* 604–612.

Lowenthal, M. F., & Robinson, B. (1976). Social networks and isolation. In R. Binstock & E. Sharns (Eds.), *Handbook of aging and the social services.* New York: Von Nostrand Reinhold.

Magarey, C. J. (1988). Aspects of the psychological management of breast cancer. *Medical Journal of Australia, 148,* 239–242.

Maguire, G. P., Lee, E. G., Bevington, D. J., Küchemann, C. S., Crabtree, R. J., & Cornell, C. E. (1978). Psychiatric problems in the first year after mastectomy. *British Medical Journal, 1,* 163–165.

Maguire, P. M. (1976). The psychological and social sequelae of mastectomy. In J. G. Howells (Ed.), *Modern perspectives in psychiatric aspects of surgery* (pp. 390–421). New York: Brunner/Mazel Publishers.

Maguire, P. M. (1978). Psychiatric problems after mastectomy. In P. C. Brand & P. A. Van Keep (Eds.), *Breast cancer: Psychosocial aspects of early detection and treatment* (pp. 47–55). Baltimore: University Park Press.

Maguire, P. M. (1983). Psychological intervention in women with breast cancer. In M. Watson & T. Morris (Eds.), *Psychological Aspects of Cancer* (pp. 77–83). Oxford: Pergamon Press.

Maguire, P. M. (1989). Breast conservation versus mastectomy: Psychological considerations. *Seminars in Surgical Oncology, 5,* 137–144.

Mailick, M. (1979). The impact of severe illness on the individual and family: An overview. *Social Work in Health Care, 5*(2), 117–128.

Malec, J., Wolberg, W., Romsaas, E., Trump, D., & Tanner, M. (1988). Million clinical multiaxial inventory (MCMI) findings among breast clinic patients after initial evaluation and at 4- or 8-month follow-up. *Journal of Clinical Psychology, 44,* 175–180.

Mann, C. (1980). Mid-life and the family: Strains, challenges and options of the middle years. In W. Norman & T. Scaramella (Eds.), *Mid-life: Developmental and clinical issues* (pp. 128–148). New York: Brunner/Mazel.

Margolis, G. J., Goodman, R. L., & Rubin, A. (1990). Psychological effects of breast-conserving cancer treatment and mastectomy. *Psychosomatics, 31,* 33–39.

Margolis, G. J., Goodman, R. L., Rubin, A., & Pajac, T. F. (1989). Psychological factors in the choice of treatment for breast cancer. *Psychosomatics, 30,* 192–197.

Markson, E. (1986). *Older women.* Lexington, MA: D. C. Heath.

McAleer, C. A., & Kluge, C. A. (1978). Counseling needs and approaches for working with a cancer patient. *Rehabilitation Counseling Bulletin, 21,* 238–245.

McArdle, C. S., Cooper, A. F., & Morran, C. (1979). The emotional and social implication of adjuvant chemotherapy in breast cancer. In S. E. Jones & S. E. Salmon (Eds.), *Adjuvant therapy of cancer* (Vol. II, *Proceedings of the second international conference.* pp. 319–325). New York: Grune & Stratton.

McCharen, N., & Earp, J. A. L. (1981). Toward a model of factors influencing the hiring of women with a history of breast cancer. *Journal of Sociology and Social Welfare, 8,* 346–363.

McCrae, R. R. (1982). Age differences in the use of coping mechanisms. *Journal of Gerontology, 37,* 454–460.

McCrae, R. R., & Costa, P. (1986). Personality, coping, and coping effectiveness in an adult sample. *Journal of Personality, 54,* 385–405.

Mercer, R., Nichols, E., & Doyle, G. C. (1989). *Transitions in a woman's life.* New York: Springer Publishing Co.

Metzger, L. F., Rogers, T. F., & Bauman, L. J. (1983). Effects of age and marital status on emotional distress after a mastectomy. *Journal of Psychosocial Oncology, 1*(3), 17–33.

Meyer, L., & Aspergren, K. (1989). Long-term psychological sequelae of mastectomy and breast conserving treatment for breast cancer. *Acta Oncologica, 28,* 13–18.

Meyerowitz, B. E. (1980). Psychosocial correlates of breast cancer and its treatments. *Psychological Bulletin, 8,* 108–131.

Meyerowitz, B. E., Chaiken, S., & Clark, L. K. (1988). Sex roles and culture: Social and personal reactions to breast cancer. In M. Fine, & A. Asch (Eds.), *Women with disabilities: Essays in psychology, culture and politics* (pp. 72–89). Philadelphia: Temple University.

Meyerowitz, B. E., Heinrich, R. L., & Coscarelli-Schag, C. (1983). A competency-based approach to coping with cancer. In T. G. Burish & L. A. Bradley (Eds.), *Coping with chronic disease: Research and applications* (pp. 137–158). Orlando: Academic Press.

Meyerowitz, B. E., Sparkes, F. C., & Spears, I. K. (1979). Psychosocial impact of adjuvant chemotherapy for breast carcinoma. *Cancer, 43,* 1613–1618.

Meyerowitz, B. E., Watkins, I. K., & Sparks, F. O. (1983). Quality of life for cancer patients receiving adjuvant chemotherapy. *American Journal of Nursing, 83,* 232–235.

Miller, J. B. (1986). *Toward a new psychology of women* (rev. ed.). Boston, MA: Beacon.

Miller, P. J. (1981). Mastectomy: A review of psychosocial research. *Health and Social Work, 6,* 60–66.

Moos, R., & Tsu, V. (1977). The crisis of physical illness: an overview. In R. Moos (Ed.), *Coping with physical illness* (pp. 3–21). New York: Plenum.

Morris, J. M. (1988). Psychosocial considerations in the surgical management of early breast cancer patients. *Dissertation Abstracts International [B], 49*(5), 1951.

Morris, T. (1979). Psychological adjustment to mastectomy. *Cancer Treatment Review, 6,* 41–61.

Morris, J., & Ingham, R. (1988). Choice of surgery for early breast cancer: Psychosocial considerations. *Social Science and Medicine, 27,* 1257–1262.

Morris, J., & Royle, G. T. (1987). Choice of surgery for early breast cancer: Pre- and postoperative levels of clinical anxiety and depression in patients and their husbands. *British Journal of Surgery, 74,* 1017–1019.

Morris, J., & Royle, G. T. (1988). Offering patients a choice of surgery for early breast cancer: A reduction in anxiety and depression in patients and their husbands. *Social Science and Medicine, 26,* 583–585.

Morris, T., Greer, S., and White, P. (1977). Psychological and social adjustment to mastectomy: A two year follow-up study. *Cancer, 40,* 2381–2387.

Nail, L., Jones, L. S., Giuffre, M., Johnson, J. E. (1984). Sensations after mastectomy. *American Journal of Nursing, 84,* 1121–1124.

National Cancer Foundation (1977). *Listen to the children: A study of the mental health of children after a parent's catastrophic illness.* New York: Cancer Care.

National Cancer Institute. (1984). *The breast cancer digest* (Report No. 84-1691). Washington, DC: National Institute of Health.

National Cancer Institute. (1985). *Cancer rates and risks.* Washington, DC: National Institute of Health.

Naysmith, A., Hinton, J. M., Meredith, R., Mackes, M. D., & Berry, R. J. (1983). Surviving malignant disease: Psychological and family aspects. *British Journal of Hospital Medicine, 30,* 22–27.

Neugarten, B. L. (1975). Adult personality: Toward a psychology of the life cycle. In W. C. Sze (Ed.), *The human life cycle.* New York: Jason Aronson.

Neugarten, B. L., & Gutmann, D. L. (1968). Age-sex roles and personality in middle age. In B. L. Neugarten (Ed.), *Middle age and aging* (pp. 58–71). Chicago: University of Chicago.

Neuling, S. J., & Winefield, H. R. (1988). Social support and recovery after surgery for breast cancer: Frequency and correlates of supportive behaviours by family, friends, and surgeon. *Social Science and Medicine, 27,* 385–392.

Newman, B. M., & Newman, P. R. (1987). *Development through life: A psychosocial approach.* Chicago, IL: Dorsey. ✳

Norman, W. H., & Scaramella, T. J. (Eds.). (1980). *Mid-life: Developmental and clinical issues.* New York: Brunner/Mazel. ✳

Northouse, L. L. (1988). Social support in patients' and husbands' adjustment to breast cancer. *Nursing Research, 37,* 91–95.

Northouse, L. L. (1989a). A longitudinal study of the adjustment of patients and husbands to breast cancer. *Oncology Nursing Forum, 16,* 511–516.

Northouse, L. L. (1989b). The impact of breast cancer on patients and husbands. *Cancer Nursing, 12,* 276–284.

Northouse, L. L., & Swain, M. A. (1987). Adjustment of patients and husbands to the initial impact of breast cancer. *Nursing Research, 36,* 221–225.

Notman, M. T. (1980). Changing roles for women at mid-life. In W. Norman & T. Scaramella (Eds.), *Mid-life: Developmental and clinical issues* (pp. 85–109). New York: Brunner/Mazel.

Novack, D. H., Plumer, R., Smith, R. L., Ochitill, H., Morrow, G. R., & Bennett, J. M. (1979). Changes in physicians' attitudes toward telling the cancer patient. *Journal of the American Medical Association, 241,* 897–900.

Nuehring, E. M., & Barr, W. E. (1980). Mastectomy: Impact on patients and families. *Health and Social Work, 5,* 51–58.

Oken, D. (1961). What to tell cancer patients: A study of medical attitudes. *Journal of the American Medical Association, 175,* 1120–1128.

Onion, P. (1981). Breast cancer: Prognosis with pregnancy. *American Journal of Nursing, 84,* 1126–1128.

Orr, E. (1986). Open communication as an effective stress management method for breast cancer patients. *Journal of Human Stress, 12,* 175–185.

Parsons, T. (1949). The social structure of the family. In R. N. Anshen (Ed.), *The family: Its function and destiny.* New York: Harper & Brothers.

Parsons, T. (1951). *The Social System.* New York: Free Press.

Parsons, T., & Fox, R. (1952). Illness, therapy, and the modern urban American family. *Journal of Social Issues, 8*(4), 31–44.

Peck, A., & Boland, J. (1977). Emotional reactions to radiation treatment. *Cancer, 40,* 180–184.

Peck, R. (1968). Psychological developments in the second half of life. In B. Neugarten (Ed.), *Middle age and aging* (pp. 88–92). Chicago, IL: University of Chicago.

Penman, D. T., Bloom, J. T., Fotopoulos, S., Cook, M. R., Holland, J. C., Gates, C., Flamer, D., Murawski, B., Ross, R., Brandt, U., Muenz, L. R., & Pee, D. (1987). The impact of mastectomy on self-concept and social function: A combined cross-sectional and longitudinal study with comparison groups. *Women and Health, 11*(3–4), 101–130.

Peters-Golden, H. (1982). Breast cancer: Varied perceptions of social support in the illness experience. *Social Science in Medicine, 16,* 483–491.

Pfeiffer, C., & Mullkien, J. B. (1984). *Caring for the patient with breast cancer.* Reston, VA: Reston.

Polivy, J. (1977). Psychological effects of mastectomy on a woman's feminine self-concept. *The Journal of Nervous and Mental Disease, 164,* 77–87.

Pollak, D. N. (1988). An assessment of women undergoing segmental mastectomy and breast irradiation for early breast cancer: Informational needs, concerns and physical sequelae. *Oncology Nursing Forum, 15,* 147.

Poole, J. (1984). Mastectomy: Its effects on interpersonal relationships. In T. O. Carlton (Ed.), *Clinical social work in health settings* (pp. 179–190). New York: Springer Publishing Co.

Psychological Aspects of Breast Cancer Study Group. (1987). Psychological response to mastectomy: A prospective comparison study. *Cancer, 59,* 189–196.

Quint, J. C. (1963). The impact of mastectomy. *American Journal of Nursing, 63,* 88–92.

Rahe, R. H. (1972). Subjects' recent life changes and their near-future illness susceptibility. *Advances in Psychosomatic Medicine, 8,* 2–19.

Ramirez, A. J., Craig, T. K., Watson, J. P., Fentiman, I. S., North, W. R., & Rubens, R. D. (1989). Stress and relapse of breast cancer. *British Medical Journal, 298* (6669), 291–293.

Reinke, B., Holmes, D., & Harris, R. (1985). The timing of psychosocial changes in women's lives: The years 25 to 45. *Journal of Marriage and the Family, 48,* 1353–1364.

Renshaw, D. C. (1983). Sex, intimacy and the older woman. *Women and Health, 8*(4), 43–54.

Riehl-Emde, A., Buddeberg, C., Muthny, F. A., Landolt-Ritter, C., Steiner, R. & Richter, D. (1989). Causal attributions and coping with illness in patients with breast cancer. *Psychotherapie Psychosomatik, Medizinische Psychologie, 39,* 232–238.

Roberts, C. S., Elkins, N. W., Baile, Jr., W. F., & Cox, C. E. (1989). Integrating research with practice: The psychosocial impact of breast cancer. *Health and Social Work, 14,* 261–268.

Roberts, P., & Newton, P. (1987). Levinsonian studies of women's adult development. *Psychology and Aging, 2,* 154–163.

Romsaas, E. P., Malec, J. F., Javenkoski, B. R., Trump, D. L., & Wolberg, W. H. (1986). Psychological distress among women with breast problems. *Cancer, 57*(4), 890–895.

Rossi, A. S. (1980). The middle years of parenting. In P. Baltos & D. G. Brim, Jr., (Eds.), *Life-span development and behavior* (Vol. 3). New York: Academic Press.

Rowland, J., Holland, J. C., Jacobs, E. R., Chaglassian, T., Geller, N., Petroni, G., Kovachev, D., & Kinne, D. (1984). Psychological response to breast reconstruction. *Continuing Medical Education Syllabus and Scientific Proceedings of the 137th Annual Meeting of the American Psychiatric Association.* Paper Sessions No. 142.

Rubin, L. (1979). *Women of a certain age: The midlife search for self.* New York: Harper & Row.

Sanger, C. L., & Reznikoff, M. (1981). A comparison of the psychological effects of breast-saving procedures with the modified radical mastectomy. *Cancer, 48*(1), 2341–2346.

Schaie, K. W., & Willis, S. L. (1986). *Adult development and aging.* Boston: Little, Brown & Company.

Schain, W. S. (1977). Psychosocial issues in counseling mastectomy patients. *The Counseling Psychologist, 6,* 45–49.

Schain, W. S. (1980). Sexual functioning, self-esteem and cancer care. *Frontiers of Radiation Therapy and Oncology, 14,* 12–19.

Schain, W. S. (1985). Breast cancer surgeries and psychosexual sequelae: Implications for remediation. *Seminars in Oncology Nursing, 1,* 200.

Schain, W. S. (1988). The sexual and intimate consequences of breast cancer treatment. *Cancer, 38,* 154–161.

Schain, W. S., Edwards, B. K., Gorrell, C. R., de Moss, E. V., Lippman, M. E., Gerber, L. H., & Lichter, A. S. (1983). Psychosocial and physical outcomes of primary breast cancer therapy: Mastectomy vs. excisional biopsy and irradiation. *Breast Cancer Research and Treatment, 3,* 377–387.

Schain, W. S., Wellisch, D. K., Pasnau, R. O., & Landsverk, J. (1985). The sooner the better: A study of psychological factors in women undergoing immediate versus delayed breast reconstruction. *American Journal of Psychiatry, 142,* 40–46.

Schlesinger, M. R., Tobin, S. S., & Kulys, R. (1980). The responsible child and parental well-being. *Journal of Gerontological Social Work, 3*(2), 3–16.

Schlossberg, N. K. (1984). *Exploring the adult years.* Washington, DC: American Psychological Association.

Schnaper, N. (1977). Psychosocial aspects of management of the patient with cancer. *Medical Clinics of North America, 61,* 1147–1155.

Schneider, J. W. & Conrad, P. (1983). *Having epilepsy: The experience and control of illness.* Philadelphia: Temple University.

Schoenrich, E. (1971). Comprehensive care for the catastrophically ill. In *Catastrophic illness in the seventies: Critical issues and complex decisions* (pp. 7–13). Proceedings of the Fourth National Symposium. New York: Cancer Care.

Schottenfeld, D., & Robbins, G. F. (1970). Quality of survival among patients who have had radical mastectomy. *Cancer, 26,* 650–654.

Schwarz, R., & Geyer, S. (1984). Social and psychological differences between cancer and noncancer patients: Cause or consequence of the disease? *Psychotherapy and Psychosomatics, 41,* 195–199.

Seltzer, V. (1988). *Every woman's guide to breast cancer.* New York: Penguin Books.

Shanas, E., & Sussman, M. B. (1979). Aging, health, and the organization of health resources. In R. W. Fogel, E. Hatfield, S. B. Kiesler, and J. March (Eds.), *Aging: stability and change in the family* (pp. 211–231). New York: Academic Press.

Sheehy, G. (1976). *Passages.* New York: Dutton.

Siegel, B. (1986). *Love, medicine, and miracles.* New York: Harper & Row.

Silberfarb, P. M., Maurer, L. H., & Crouthamel, C. S. (1980). Psychosocial aspects of neoplastic disease: Functional status of breast cancer patients during different treatment regimens. *American Journal of Psychiatry, 137,* 450–455.

Sinsheimer, L. M., & Holland, J. C. (1987). Psychological issues in breast cancer. *Seminars in Oncology 14*, 75–82.

Smith, E. M., Redman, R., Burns, T. L., & Sagert, K. M. (1985). Perceptions of social support among patients with recently diagnosed breast, endometrial, and ovarian cancer: An exploratory study. *Journal of Psychosocial Oncology, 3*, 65–81.

Spiegel, D., Bloom, J. R., Kraemer, H. C., & Gottheil, E. (1989). Effect of psychosocial treatment on survival of patients with metastatic breast cancer. *Lancet, 2* (8668), 888–891.

Starr, B., & Weiner, M. (1981) *The Starr-Weiner report on sex and sexuality in the mature years*. New York: McGraw-Hill.

Steger, H. G. (1977). Trauma in the young adult. In E. M. Pattison (Ed.), *The experience of dying* (pp. 213–225). Englewood Cliffs, NJ: Prentice Hall.

Steinberg, M. D., Juliano, M. A., & Wise, L. (1985). Psychological outcome of lumpectomy versus mastectomy in the treatment of breast cancer. *American Journal of Psychiatry, 142*, 34–39.

Stewart, W. (1977). A psychosocial study of the formation of the early adult life structure in women (Doctoral dissertation, Columbia University, 1976). *Dissertation Abstracts International, 38*, 1B.

Stueve, A., & O'Donnell, L. (1984). The daughter of aging parents. In G. Baruch & J. Brooks-Gunn (Eds.), *Women in midlife* (pp. 203–225). New York: Plenum.

Taylor, S. E., Lichtman, R. R., Wood, J. V., Bluming, A. Z., Dosik, G. M., & Liebowitz, R. L. (1985). Illness-related treatment-related factors in psychological adjustment to breast cancer. *Cancer, 55*, 2506–2513.

Thomas, S. G. (1978). Breast cancer: The psychosocial issues. *Cancer Nursing, 1*, 53–60.

Tish-Knobf, M. K. (1984). CE breast cancer: The treatment revolution. *American Journal of Nursing, 84*, 1110–1120.

Tish-Knobf, M. K. (1986). Physical and psychologic distress associated with adjuvant chemotherapy in women with breast cancer. *Journal of Clinical Oncology, 4*, 678–684.

Troll, L. E. (1982). Family life in middle and old age: The generation gap. *The Annals of the American Academy of Political and Social Science, 464*, 38–46.

Tross, S. (1989). Psychological sequelae in cancer survivors. In J. C. Holland & J. H. Rowland (Eds.), *Handbook of psychooncology: Psychological care of the cancer patient*. New York: Oxford.

Turner, F. J. (Ed.). (1984). *Adult psychopathology: A social work perspective*. New York: Macmillan.

U.S. Senate Special Committee on Aging. (1981). *Developments in aging: 1981*. Washington, DC: U.S. Government Printing Office.

Vachon, M. L. S., Lyall, W. A. L., & Freeman, S. J. J. (1978). Measurement and management of stress in health professionals working with advanced cancer patients. *Death Education, 1*, 365–375.

Vinokur, A. D., Threatt, B. A., Caplan, R. D., & Zimmerman, B. L. (1989). Physical and psychosocial functioning and adjustment to breast cancer. *Cancer, 63*, 394–405.

Walker, A., Pratt, C., Shin, H. Y., & Jones, L. (1990). Motives for parental caregiving and relationship quality. *Family Relations, 39,* 51–56.

Walter, C. A. (1988, March). *Mothers and daughters: Understanding powerful dynamics in the caregiving relationship.* Paper presented at the 34th Annual Meeting, American Society on Aging, San Diego, Calif.

Walter, C. A. (1989, October). *Adult daughters and mothers: Stress in the caregiving relationship.* Paper presented at the annual meeting of the National Association of Social Workers, San Francisco, CA.

Weick, A. (1983). A growth-task model of human development. *Social Casework, 64,* 131–137.

Weisman, A. D. (1976). Early diagnosis of vulnerability in cancer patients. *American Journal of Medical Sciences, 271,* 187–196.

Weisman, A. D., & Worden, J. W. (1977). *Coping and vulnerability in cancer patients: A research report.* Cambridge, MA: Project Omega, Department of Psychiatry, Harvard Medical School, Massachusetts General Hospital.

Wellisch, D. K. (1979). Adolescent acting out when a parent has cancer. *International Journal of Family Therapy, 1,* 230.

Wellisch, D. K. (1985). The psychologic impact of breast cancer on relationships. *Seminars in Oncology Nursing, 1,* 195–199.

Wellisch, D. K., Jamison, K. R., & Pasnaw, R. O. (1978). Psychological aspects of mastectomy: 2. The man's perspective. *American Journal of Psychiatry, 135,* 543–546.

Wellisch, D. K., Landsverk, J., Guidera, K., Pasnau, R. O., & Fawzy, F. (1983). Evaluation of psychosocial problems of the homebound cancer patient: Methodology and problem frequencies. *Psychosomatic Medicine, 45,* 11–21.

Wellisch, D. K., Schain, W. S., Noone, R. B., & Little, J. W. (1987). The psychological contribution of nipple addition in breast reconstruction. *Plastic and Reconstructive Surgery, 80,* 699–704.

Wiener, C. L. (1975). The burden of rheumatoid arthritis. In A. L. Strauss and B. G. Glaser (Eds.), *Chronic illness and the quality of life* (pp. 71–80). St. Louis: Mosby.

Wise, T. N. (1978). Sexual functioning in neoplastic disease. *Medical Aspects of Human Sexuality, 12,* 16–31.

Wissing, V. S. (1984). The hormone factor. *American Journal of Nursing, 84,* 1117–1119.

Witkin, M. H. (1975). Sex therapy and mastectomy. *Journal of Sex Therapy and Marital Therapy, 1,* 290–304.

Witkin, M. H. (1979). Psychological concerns in sexual rehabilitation and mastectomy. *Sexuality and Disability, 2,* 54–59.

Wolberg, W. H., Romsaas, E. P., Tanner, M. A., & Malec, J. F. (1989). Psychosexual adaptation to breast cancer surgery. *Cancer, 63,* 1645–1655.

Wolberg, W. H., Tanner, M. A., Romsaas, E. P., Trump, D. L., & Malec, J. F. (1987). Factors influencing options in primary breast cancer treatment. *Journal of Clinical Oncology, 5,* 68–74.

Woods, N. (1979). *Human sexuality in health and illness.* St. Louis: Mosby.

Woods, N., & Earp, J. (1978). Women with cured breast cancer: A study of mastectomy patients in North Carolina. *Nursing Research, 27,* 279–285.

Worden, J. W., & Weisman, A. D. (1977). The fallacy in postmastectomy depression. *American Journal of the Medical Sciences, 273,* 169–175.

Worden, J. W., & Weisman, A. D. (1985). Psychosocial components of lagtime in cancer diagnosis. *Journal of Psychosomatic Research, 19,* 69–79.

Wortman, C. B., & Dunkel-Schetter, C. (1979). Interpersonal relationships and cancer: A theoretical analysis. *Journal of Social Issues, 35*(1), 120–155.

Young-Eisendrath, P. (1984). Demeter's folly: Experiencing loss in middle life. *Psychological Perspectives, 15,* 39–63.

Zastrow, C., & Kirst-Ashman. (1987). *Understanding human behavior and the social environment.* Chicago, IL: Nelson-Hall.

Zemore, R., & Shepel, L. F. (1989). Effects of breast cancer and mastectomy on emotional support and adjustment. *Social Science and Medicine, 28,* 19–27.

Index

Index